Menopause Galveston Diet Cookbook

Restore Hormonal Balance Through Targeted Nutrition and the Right Anti-inflammatory Approach. Easy and Delicious Recipes, Without Compromises

Marie Dowson

© **Copyright 2024 by Marie Dowson - All rights reserved.**

The following book is provided below with the aim of delivering information that is as precise and dependable as possible. However, purchasing this book implies an acknowledgment that both the publisher and the author are not experts in the discussed topics, and any recommendations or suggestions contained herein are solely for entertainment purposes. It is advised that professionals be consulted as needed before acting on any endorsed actions.

This statement is considered fair and valid by both the American Bar Association and the Committee of Publishers Association, and it holds legal binding throughout the United States.

Moreover, any transmission, duplication, or reproduction of this work, including specific information, will be deemed an illegal act, regardless of whether it is done electronically or in print. This includes creating secondary or tertiary copies of the work or recorded copies, which are only allowed with the express written consent from the Publisher. All additional rights are reserved.

The information in the following pages is generally considered to be a truthful and accurate account of facts. As such, any negligence, use, or misuse of the information by the reader will result in actions falling solely under their responsibility. There are no scenarios in which the publisher or the original author can be held liable for any difficulties or damages that may occur after undertaking the information described herein.

Additionally, the information in the following pages is intended solely for informational purposes and should be considered as such. As fitting its nature, it is presented without assurance regarding its prolonged validity or interim quality. Mention of trademarks is done without written consent and should not be construed as an endorsement from the trademark holder.

TABLE OF CONTENTS

CHAPTER 1: GALVESTON LIFESTYLE 7

1. Understanding the Galveston Diet 7
Key Principles and Benefits 7
Comparison with Other Diets 9
Scientific Backing and Research 11

2. Daily Routines for Success 14
Structuring Your Day Around the Diet 14
Meal Timing and Frequency 16
Incorporating Exercise and Physical Activity 19

3. Creating a Supportive Environment 21
Stocking Your Kitchen with Essentials 21
Managing Social Situations and Eating Out 23
Building a Support Network 25

4. Adapting the Lifestyle to Fit Your Needs 28
Customizing the Diet for Different Lifestyles 28

CHAPTER 2: MINDSET AND GOALS 31

1. Setting Realistic and Achievable Goals 31
Defining Your Personal Objectives 31
Short-Term vs. Long-Term Goals 33
Measuring Success and Progress 35

2. Cultivating a Positive Mindset 38
Overcoming Negative Self-Talk 38
Developing Resilience and Patience 40
Techniques for Staying Motivated 42

CHAPTER 3: BREAKFASTS 45

CHAPTER 4: LUNCHES 51

CHAPTER 5: DINNERS 57

CHAPTER 6: SNACKS AND SIDES 63

CHAPTER 7: DESSERTS 69

CHAPTER 8: REFRESHING BEVERAGES 75

CHAPTER 9: FISH AND SEAFOOD DELIGHTS 81

CHAPTER 10: POULTRY AND BEEF FAVORITES 87

CHAPTER 11: FRESH AND FLAVORFUL SALADS 93

CHAPTER 12: DELICIOUS VEGETARIAN OPTIONS 99

CHAPTER 13: HEARTY SOUPS AND STEWS 107

CHAPTER 14: WHAT TO EAT WHEN YOU'RE OUT 117

28 DAYS EASY MEAL PLAN 119

CHAPTER 1: GALVESTON LIFESTYLE

1. UNDERSTANDING THE GALVESTON DIET

KEY PRINCIPLES AND BENEFITS

The Galveston Diet is not just another diet plan; it's a lifestyle designed to bring balance and vitality during a transformative phase of life—menopause. Understanding its key principles and the benefits it offers can be the cornerstone of a journey toward better health and well-being.

At its core, the Galveston Diet emphasizes an anti-inflammatory approach to eating. This focus is particularly beneficial during menopause, a time when hormonal fluctuations can lead to increased inflammation in the body. Inflammation is linked to a host of health issues, including weight gain, fatigue, joint pain, and even chronic conditions like heart disease and diabetes. By prioritizing anti-inflammatory foods, the Galveston Diet aims to mitigate these risks and promote overall wellness.

A significant principle of the Galveston Diet is its emphasis on nutrient-dense, whole foods. Unlike many restrictive diets that cut out entire food groups or severely limit caloric intake, the Galveston Diet encourages the consumption of a variety of fruits, vegetables, lean proteins, and healthy fats. These foods are not only rich in essential nutrients but also help to stabilize blood sugar levels, reduce cravings, and maintain energy throughout the day.

Protein plays a pivotal role in the Galveston Diet. As women age, maintaining muscle mass becomes increasingly important, not only for strength and mobility but also for metabolic health. Lean proteins, such as fish, poultry, legumes, and nuts, are integral to the diet, helping to support muscle repair and growth, which is crucial for a healthy metabolism and overall vitality.

Healthy fats are another cornerstone of the Galveston Diet. Far from the outdated notion that all fats are detrimental, this diet recognizes the importance of incorporating healthy fats from sources like avocados, olive oil, nuts, and seeds. These fats are vital for hormone production, brain health, and satiety. They also play a crucial role in reducing inflammation, a key goal of the diet.

Carbohydrates in the Galveston Diet are carefully chosen to support health and well-being. Instead of refined carbs that can spike blood sugar and contribute to inflammation, the diet focuses on complex carbs found in whole grains, vegetables, and fruits. These carbs provide sustained energy and are packed with fiber, which aids in digestion and helps to maintain a healthy gut microbiome.

Intermittent fasting is another important aspect of the Galveston Diet. This eating pattern involves alternating periods of eating and fasting, which can help to balance insulin levels, support metabolic health, and promote fat loss. By giving the body regular breaks from food intake, intermittent fasting can help to reduce inflammation and improve cellular repair processes, making it a powerful tool for enhancing overall health during menopause.

Hydration is a simple yet often overlooked principle of the Galveston Diet. Staying adequately hydrated is essential for all bodily functions, including digestion, circulation, and temperature regulation. Drinking plenty of water helps to flush out toxins, keep skin healthy, and maintain energy levels. The Galveston Diet encourages drinking water throughout the day and limiting sugary beverages, which can contribute to inflammation and weight gain.

One of the key benefits of the Galveston Diet is its adaptability to individual needs and preferences. This flexibility is crucial, especially during menopause, when every woman's experience can be different. The diet can be tailored to accommodate various dietary restrictions and preferences, ensuring that it is sustainable and enjoyable for the long term. Whether you are vegetarian, gluten-free, or have other specific dietary needs, the Galveston Diet can be customized to suit your lifestyle.

Moreover, the Galveston Diet is supported by scientific research, which adds to its credibility and effectiveness. Studies have shown that anti-inflammatory diets can help to reduce symptoms associated with menopause, such as hot flashes, mood swings, and sleep disturbances. By focusing on nutrient-dense, anti-inflammatory foods, the Galveston Diet provides a balanced approach that not only addresses menopausal symptoms but also supports overall health and longevity.

Another important benefit of the Galveston Diet is its potential to support weight management. Weight gain during menopause is a common concern, often exacerbated by hormonal changes that affect metabolism and fat distribution. The Galveston Diet's emphasis on whole foods, healthy fats, and intermittent fasting helps to regulate blood sugar levels and support metabolic health, making it easier to manage weight during this stage of life. This approach not only aids in shedding excess pounds but also helps to prevent weight-related health issues, such as type 2 diabetes and cardiovascular disease.

In addition to physical health benefits, the Galveston Diet also promotes mental and emotional well-being. The diet's focus on balanced nutrition and stable blood sugar levels can help to improve mood and reduce anxiety and depression, which are common during menopause. Furthermore, the diet encourages a mindful approach to eating, fostering a positive relationship with food and promoting self-care. This holistic approach is essential for overall wellness, helping women to feel empowered and in control of their health.

The Galveston Diet also recognizes the importance of community and support. Navigating menopause can be challenging, and having a supportive network can make a significant difference. The diet encourages building a support system, whether it's through family, friends, or online communities. Sharing experiences, tips, and recipes can provide motivation and encouragement, making the journey toward better health more enjoyable and sustainable.

Ultimately, the Galveston Diet is about creating a sustainable, healthy lifestyle that supports hormonal balance and overall well-being during menopause. By focusing on anti-inflammatory, nutrient-dense foods, healthy fats, lean proteins, and mindful eating practices, the diet provides a comprehensive approach to managing menopausal symptoms and improving health. The adaptability and scientific backing of the diet make it a credible and effective option for women seeking to enhance their quality of life during this transformative phase.

In conclusion, the Galveston Diet offers a balanced, holistic approach to nutrition and lifestyle that addresses the unique challenges of menopause. Its emphasis on anti-inflammatory foods, intermittent fasting, and personalized nutrition provides a solid foundation for managing symptoms and promoting long-term health. By understanding and embracing the key principles and benefits of the Galveston Diet, women can take proactive steps toward achieving hormonal balance and overall well-being, making the journey through menopause a positive and empowering experience.

COMPARISON WITH OTHER DIETS

When exploring the landscape of diets available today, the Galveston Diet stands out with its unique focus on menopausal women's needs. To truly appreciate its value, it's helpful to compare it with some of the more popular diets: the Mediterranean Diet, the Keto Diet, and the Paleo Diet. Each of these diets has its merits and principles, but the Galveston Diet brings a distinct approach tailored to the hormonal changes and specific health concerns of menopause.

The Mediterranean Diet, hailed for its heart-healthy benefits, emphasizes fruits, vegetables, whole grains, and healthy fats, primarily from olive oil. Fish and poultry are favored over red meat, and there's a modest intake of dairy. The Mediterranean Diet promotes moderate consumption of wine, typically with meals, reflecting the dietary patterns of countries bordering the Mediterranean Sea. It's known for its anti-inflammatory properties, which align with the principles of the Galveston Diet. However, the Galveston Diet takes this a step further by specifically addressing the nutritional needs during menopause, emphasizing foods that support hormonal balance and metabolic health. For instance, while both diets advocate for healthy fats, the Galveston Diet specifically encourages sources that aid in hormone production, such as avocados and seeds, which can be particularly beneficial for women in menopause.

On the other hand, the Keto Diet focuses on a high-fat, low-carbohydrate regimen designed to shift the body into a state of ketosis, where it burns fat for fuel instead of carbohydrates. This diet can lead to significant weight loss and improved blood sugar control. However, its stringent restrictions on carbohydrate intake often mean that whole grains, fruits, and many vegetables are limited, which can be challenging to maintain and might not provide the comprehensive nutrient profile necessary for overall health. The Galveston Diet, while also reducing refined carbohydrates, maintains a balanced approach by including complex carbs like whole grains and vegetables that are essential for sustained energy and digestive health. This balance is particularly important during menopause, when nutritional needs are heightened, and the risk of bone density loss and other health concerns increases.

The Paleo Diet, often referred to as the "caveman diet," promotes eating foods that were available to our Paleolithic ancestors. This means a focus on meats, fish, fruits, vegetables, nuts, and seeds, while excluding dairy, grains, and processed foods. The idea is to eat in a way that is aligned with human genetics and avoid the processed foods that are prevalent in modern diets. While the Paleo Diet shares the Galveston Diet's emphasis on whole, unprocessed foods, it can be overly restrictive and may not address the specific needs of menopausal women. The exclusion of whole grains and legumes in the Paleo Diet can lead to a lack of important nutrients and fiber, which are crucial for digestive health and hormonal balance. The Galveston Diet, by contrast, allows for a more varied intake of nutrient-dense foods, ensuring a more comprehensive nutritional approach that supports overall health and wellness during menopause.

Another comparison worth making is with the DASH Diet (Dietary Approaches to Stop Hypertension), which is designed to reduce blood pressure and promote heart health. It emphasizes fruits, vegetables, whole grains, lean proteins, and low-fat dairy, while reducing salt, red meat, and sweets. While the DASH Diet's focus on reducing hypertension is beneficial, it doesn't specifically cater to the hormonal fluctuations and metabolic changes associated with menopause. The Galveston Diet's tailored approach includes not only the anti-inflammatory foods that support cardiovascular health but also specific strategies like intermittent fasting to help manage weight and insulin sensitivity, issues that can be particularly challenging during menopause.

The intermittent fasting component of the Galveston Diet sets it apart from many other diets. Intermittent fasting involves cycling between periods of eating and fasting, which can help regulate insulin levels, improve metabolic health, and promote fat loss. While some diets might focus solely on what to eat, the Galveston Diet also addresses when to eat, providing a holistic approach that can be particularly effective for managing weight and health during menopause. This aspect is designed to fit seamlessly into a busy lifestyle, offering flexibility and simplicity, which can be appealing to many women juggling various responsibilities.

Moreover, the Galveston Diet's specific focus on anti-inflammatory foods is particularly relevant during menopause. Inflammation is a common issue due to hormonal changes, and managing it can alleviate many menopausal symptoms such as joint pain, fatigue, and mood swings. While the Mediterranean and DASH diets also emphasize anti-inflammatory foods, the Galveston Diet uniquely combines this with hormonal balance strategies, providing a dual approach that targets the root causes of many menopausal symptoms.

Another noteworthy aspect is the Galveston Diet's inclusivity and adaptability. Unlike the Paleo or Keto diets, which can be quite rigid, the Galveston Diet offers flexibility, allowing women to tailor the diet to their individual needs and preferences. This can make it easier to adhere to in the long term, promoting sustained health benefits. The diet encourages a mindful approach to eating, emphasizing the importance of listening to one's body and making adjustments as needed, which is particularly empowering for women navigating the changes of menopause.

The Galveston Diet also emphasizes the importance of building a supportive community, recognizing that lifestyle changes are more successful when shared with others. Whether through online communities, family, or friends, having a network of support can provide motivation, encouragement, and accountability. This social aspect is often overlooked in other diets but is integral to the Galveston Diet, helping women to stay committed and enjoy the journey toward better health.

In summary, while each of these popular diets—the Mediterranean, Keto, Paleo, and DASH—has its benefits, the Galveston Diet offers a uniquely comprehensive approach tailored to the needs of menopausal women. Its emphasis on anti-inflammatory, nutrient-dense foods, balanced with healthy fats and lean proteins, and its inclusion of intermittent fasting, provide a robust framework for managing menopausal symptoms and promoting overall health. The flexibility and adaptability of the diet, combined with its focus on community support and mindfulness, make it not just a diet but a sustainable lifestyle change. This holistic approach ensures that women can navigate menopause with confidence, vitality, and a renewed sense of well-being.

SCIENTIFIC BACKING AND RESEARCH

The scientific backing of the Galveston Diet is both extensive and compelling, providing a strong foundation for its principles and practices. Understanding this research not only enhances the credibility of the diet but also offers reassurance and confidence to those embarking on this journey toward better health and hormonal balance during menopause.

The core of the Galveston Diet lies in its anti-inflammatory approach. Inflammation is a natural immune response, but chronic inflammation is linked to numerous health problems, including heart disease, diabetes, and various autoimmune conditions. For menopausal women, inflammation can exacerbate symptoms such as joint pain, fatigue, and hot flashes.

Studies have shown that diets rich in anti-inflammatory foods, such as fruits, vegetables, nuts, and seeds, can significantly reduce these issues. Research published in the journal *Nature Medicine* highlights the benefits of such diets in reducing inflammatory markers in the body, which can alleviate symptoms and improve overall health.

One of the key components of the Galveston Diet is the emphasis on healthy fats, particularly those found in sources like olive oil, avocados, and fatty fish. These fats are essential for hormone production and brain health, which are crucial during menopause. Omega-3 fatty acids, abundant in fatty fish, have been shown to reduce inflammation and improve mood and cognitive function. A study published in the *American Journal of Clinical Nutrition* demonstrated that omega-3 supplementation significantly reduced the frequency and severity of hot flashes and night sweats in menopausal women. This underscores the importance of incorporating healthy fats into the diet to manage menopausal symptoms effectively.

Protein intake is another critical aspect of the Galveston Diet. As women age, maintaining muscle mass becomes increasingly important for metabolic health and physical function. Research indicates that adequate protein intake helps preserve muscle mass and strength, reducing the risk of sarcopenia (age-related muscle loss). A study in the *Journal of Nutrition* found that higher protein consumption was associated with greater muscle mass and lower body fat in older adults. This evidence supports the Galveston Diet's recommendation to include lean proteins such as poultry, fish, legumes, and nuts, which not only aid in muscle maintenance but also provide essential nutrients for overall health.

Intermittent fasting, a practice incorporated into the Galveston Diet, has garnered significant scientific interest for its potential health benefits. Intermittent fasting involves alternating periods of eating and fasting, which can help regulate insulin levels, enhance metabolic health, and promote fat loss. Research published in the *New England Journal of Medicine* highlights the various benefits of intermittent fasting, including improved insulin sensitivity, reduced inflammation, and enhanced cellular repair processes. These effects are particularly beneficial for menopausal women, who often face challenges related to insulin resistance and weight gain.

Hydration is a simple yet crucial component of the Galveston Diet, supported by scientific evidence. Adequate hydration is essential for all bodily functions, including digestion, circulation, and temperature regulation. Research indicates that proper hydration can improve energy levels, cognitive function, and skin health. A study in the journal *Nutrition Reviews* found that even mild dehydration can impair mood and cognitive performance, emphasizing the importance of drinking sufficient water throughout the day. The Galveston Diet's focus on whole, unprocessed foods is also backed by extensive research.

Diets high in processed foods are linked to increased inflammation, weight gain, and a higher risk of chronic diseases. Conversely, whole foods provide essential nutrients, fiber, and antioxidants that support overall health. A study in *The Lancet* demonstrated that diets rich in fruits, vegetables, whole grains, and nuts are associated with a lower risk of mortality from cardiovascular disease and cancer. This evidence reinforces the Galveston Diet's emphasis on whole, nutrient-dense foods as a cornerstone of health and longevity.

Fiber intake, emphasized in the Galveston Diet through the inclusion of fruits, vegetables, and whole grains, plays a vital role in digestive health and hormonal balance. Fiber supports a healthy gut microbiome, which is crucial for nutrient absorption and immune function. Research published in the journal *Gut* highlights the connection between a high-fiber diet and reduced inflammation, as well as improved gut health. Additionally, fiber helps regulate blood sugar levels, which can be particularly beneficial for managing weight and reducing the risk of type 2 diabetes, a concern for many women during menopause.

Another important aspect of the Galveston Diet is its adaptability to individual needs and preferences, which is crucial for long-term adherence and success. Research indicates that personalized nutrition approaches are more effective in promoting sustainable dietary changes and improving health outcomes. A study in the journal *Cell Metabolism* found that individualized dietary recommendations based on genetic, metabolic, and microbiome data led to better compliance and health improvements compared to generic dietary guidelines. This supports the Galveston Diet's flexible approach, allowing women to tailor the diet to their unique needs and preferences while still adhering to its core principles.

The scientific evidence also supports the psychological and emotional benefits of the Galveston Diet. A nutrient-rich, balanced diet can have a profound impact on mental health, reducing symptoms of anxiety and depression that are common during menopause. Research published in *The American Journal of Psychiatry* found that a healthy diet, rich in fruits, vegetables, whole grains, and lean proteins, was associated with a lower risk of depression. This underscores the importance of the Galveston Diet's holistic approach, which not only addresses physical health but also promotes mental and emotional well-being.

In addition to the nutritional components, the Galveston Diet encourages regular physical activity, which is supported by extensive research for its health benefits. Exercise helps maintain muscle mass, supports cardiovascular health, and improves mood and energy levels. A study in *The Journal of Clinical Endocrinology & Metabolism* found that regular exercise significantly improved menopausal symptoms, including hot flashes, sleep disturbances, and mood swings. This evidence aligns with the Galveston Diet's recommendation to incorporate physical activity as part of a healthy lifestyle. Furthermore, the Galveston Diet's emphasis on a supportive community is backed by research highlighting the importance of social connections for health and well-being. Studies have shown that individuals who have strong social support networks are more likely to adhere to healthy behaviors and experience better health outcomes. Research published in the journal *Health Psychology* found that social support was associated with improved adherence to dietary and exercise recommendations, as well as better mental health. This reinforces the value of building a support network as part of the Galveston Diet, helping women to stay motivated and connected on their health journey.

In conclusion, the scientific backing and research supporting the Galveston Diet are robust and compelling. The diet's principles are grounded in extensive evidence, demonstrating the benefits of an anti-inflammatory approach, healthy fats, adequate protein, intermittent fasting, hydration, whole foods, and personalized nutrition. This comprehensive approach not only addresses the unique challenges of menopause but also promotes overall health and well-being. By understanding and embracing the scientific foundations of the Galveston Diet, women can make informed choices that support their health and vitality during this transformative phase of life.

2. Daily Routines for Success

Structuring Your Day Around the Diet

Embracing the Galveston Diet isn't just about what you eat—it's about how you integrate its principles into your daily life. Structuring your day around the diet can create a seamless flow that maximizes the benefits of this balanced, anti-inflammatory approach to nutrition, particularly during menopause. Let's walk through a typical day, envisioning how to weave the Galveston Diet into your routine in a way that feels natural and sustainable.

Imagine waking up to a new day, the early morning light filtering through your bedroom window. You start with a gentle stretch, appreciating the quiet moments before the bustle begins. Hydration is key first thing in the morning. A glass of water infused with a slice of lemon can jumpstart your metabolism and begin the day with a refreshing note. The lemon not only adds a pleasant flavor but also provides a gentle dose of vitamin C, an antioxidant that supports your immune system and skin health.

As you move into your morning routine, think about breakfast. This meal sets the tone for the day, providing the energy and nutrients your body needs after a night of fasting. The Galveston Diet emphasizes balanced meals, so consider something that combines protein, healthy fats, and fiber. For example, you might enjoy a bowl of Greek yogurt topped with fresh berries and a sprinkle of chia seeds.

The yogurt provides protein and probiotics for gut health, the berries add antioxidants and fiber, and the chia seeds offer omega-3 fatty acids and more fiber, keeping you satisfied and energized.

Mornings can be busy, whether you're heading to work, exercising, or managing household tasks. Keeping a nutritious snack on hand can help maintain your energy levels and prevent the temptation of less healthy options. Nuts and seeds are excellent choices, offering a good balance of protein and healthy fats. A small handful of almonds or pumpkin seeds can be easily packed in your bag or kept in your desk drawer.

Lunch should be another balanced affair, focusing on anti-inflammatory foods that sustain your energy for the rest of the day. A vibrant salad with a variety of colorful vegetables, a source of lean protein like grilled chicken or chickpeas, and a dressing made from olive oil and lemon juice can be both satisfying and nutrient-dense. The vegetables provide a range of vitamins and minerals, the protein helps with muscle maintenance and satiety, and the olive oil dressing offers healthy fats that support heart and brain health.

Afternoons might bring a slump in energy, a common experience for many. Instead of reaching for a sugary snack or caffeine, consider a cup of green tea. Green tea contains antioxidants and a moderate amount of caffeine, providing a gentle energy boost without the crash. Pair it with a piece of fruit, like an apple or a handful of berries, to satisfy your sweet tooth naturally while also providing fiber and nutrients.

Dinner on the Galveston Diet should be a relaxing and fulfilling experience, a time to unwind and nourish your body with wholesome foods. Think about including a variety of vegetables, a source of lean protein, and a serving of healthy fats. Perhaps you could enjoy a piece of salmon, rich in omega-3 fatty acids, alongside roasted vegetables like Brussels sprouts and sweet potatoes. The salmon supports brain and heart health, the Brussels sprouts offer fiber and antioxidants, and the sweet potatoes provide a good source of complex carbohydrates and vitamins.

Evening routines often include winding down and preparing for rest. Hydration remains important throughout the day, so consider ending your evening with a calming herbal tea. Chamomile or peppermint tea can aid in digestion and promote relaxation, helping to prepare your body for a good night's sleep.

Incorporating intermittent fasting into your daily routine is another way to enhance the benefits of the Galveston Diet. This might mean finishing your dinner by 7 PM and not eating again until 11 AM the next day. This fasting period allows your body to reset and repair, supporting metabolic health and reducing inflammation. If intermittent fasting feels challenging at first, try gradually increasing the fasting window by an hour each day until you reach a duration that feels comfortable and sustainable.

Physical activity is another integral part of structuring your day around the Galveston Diet. Aim to include some form of exercise, whether it's a morning walk, a yoga session, or an evening bike ride. Exercise complements the diet by supporting cardiovascular health, maintaining muscle mass, and boosting mood through the release of endorphins. Find activities that you enjoy and look forward to, making them a regular part of your routine.

Social connections and support can also play a significant role in your success with the Galveston Diet. Consider sharing meals with family or friends, joining a community group, or participating in online forums where you can exchange tips, recipes, and encouragement. Building a supportive network helps maintain motivation and can make the journey more enjoyable and less isolating.

Mindfulness and stress management are equally important. Practicing mindfulness through meditation, deep breathing exercises, or simply taking a few moments of quiet reflection can help reduce stress and improve your overall well-being. Chronic stress can exacerbate inflammation and negatively impact hormonal balance, so incorporating these practices can have a profound effect on your health.

As the day comes to a close, reflect on how you felt. Did you have steady energy throughout the day? Were your meals satisfying and enjoyable? Listening to your body's responses can guide adjustments, ensuring that the Galveston Diet becomes a seamless and rewarding part of your daily life.

Structuring your day around the Galveston Diet involves more than just meal planning; it's about creating a balanced, mindful lifestyle that supports your health and well-being during menopause. By incorporating nutrient-dense foods, staying hydrated, engaging in regular physical activity, and practicing mindfulness, you can navigate this transformative phase with vitality and confidence. Each day is an opportunity to nourish your body and mind, fostering a sense of empowerment and well-being that extends far beyond the kitchen.

MEAL TIMING AND FREQUENCY

One of the most crucial aspects of the Galveston Diet is understanding meal timing and frequency. These factors play a significant role in how your body processes nutrients, manages hunger, and maintains energy levels throughout the day. By strategically planning when and how often you eat, you can optimize your health, particularly during menopause.

Imagine waking up in the morning with the dawn of a new day. Your body has been fasting overnight, giving it time to rest, repair, and reset. This natural fasting period is extended and supported by the Galveston Diet's approach to intermittent fasting. Instead of diving straight into breakfast, you might start your day with a glass of water, allowing your body to wake up gradually.

This period of hydration sets the stage for a mindful eating pattern that aligns with your body's rhythms.

The concept of intermittent fasting, which is integral to the Galveston Diet, involves cycling between periods of eating and fasting. A common pattern is the 16:8 method, where you fast for 16 hours and eat during an 8-hour window. For example, you might finish dinner by 7 PM and not eat again until 11 AM the next day. This fasting window gives your body ample time to digest the previous day's food, lower insulin levels, and initiate cellular repair processes. Research has shown that intermittent fasting can help regulate insulin sensitivity, promote weight loss, and reduce inflammation, all of which are particularly beneficial during menopause.

When it's time for your first meal, think of it as breaking the fast. This meal should be balanced and nourishing, providing the right blend of protein, healthy fats, and fiber to kickstart your metabolism and keep you feeling full and energized. Consider how you might savor a bowl of oatmeal topped with fresh berries and a dollop of almond butter. The oats offer complex carbohydrates and fiber, the berries provide antioxidants and vitamins, and the almond butter adds healthy fats and protein. This combination helps to stabilize blood sugar levels, which is essential for managing energy and mood throughout the day.

As the morning progresses, listen to your body's hunger signals. The Galveston Diet encourages mindful eating, which means paying attention to when you're truly hungry versus eating out of habit or boredom. This mindfulness can help you avoid unnecessary snacking and make more deliberate choices. If you find yourself needing a mid-morning snack, opt for something light and nutritious, like a handful of nuts or a piece of fruit. These options provide a good balance of macronutrients without spiking your blood sugar.

Lunchtime should be another opportunity to refuel with nutrient-dense foods. Picture a vibrant salad filled with leafy greens, colorful vegetables, a source of lean protein such as grilled chicken or tofu, and a healthy fat like avocado or olive oil. This meal not only provides a variety of vitamins and minerals but also supports sustained energy levels. The fiber in the vegetables aids digestion, the protein helps maintain muscle mass, and the healthy fats are crucial for hormone production and brain health.

In the afternoon, you might experience a natural dip in energy. Instead of reaching for a sugary snack or caffeine, which can lead to energy crashes later, consider a balanced snack that includes protein and healthy fats. A small serving of Greek yogurt with a sprinkle of nuts or seeds can be a satisfying option. This snack supports your body's needs without overwhelming it with excess calories or sugar. Dinner is an important meal that should be consumed at a reasonable hour, ideally a few hours before bedtime.

This allows your body to digest the meal properly before you go to sleep. Think about a dinner plate filled with a variety of roasted vegetables, a portion of lean protein like salmon or legumes, and a serving of whole grains such as quinoa or brown rice. This meal structure supports the Galveston Diet's principles by providing a balanced array of nutrients that promote satiety and nourishment.

As the evening winds down, hydration remains key. Drinking a calming herbal tea can help you relax and prepare for a good night's sleep. Chamomile or peppermint tea are excellent choices that aid digestion and promote relaxation. Avoid late-night snacking, as it can disrupt your digestive processes and interfere with the benefits of intermittent fasting.

One of the beautiful aspects of meal timing and frequency within the Galveston Diet is its adaptability. While the 16:8 intermittent fasting pattern is common, it's important to find what works best for your body and lifestyle. Some might prefer a 14:10 or even a 12:12 fasting-to-eating ratio. The key is to create a consistent routine that your body can adapt to, promoting regularity and balance.

Integrating meal timing with your daily activities is also crucial. For instance, if you exercise regularly, plan your meals around your workouts to maximize energy and recovery. Eating a balanced meal after a workout can replenish glycogen stores and support muscle repair. Similarly, if you have a busy day ahead, ensure your meals are planned and prepared in advance to avoid the temptation of less healthy convenience foods.

The benefits of structured meal timing and frequency go beyond physical health; they also support mental and emotional well-being. Regular meals and mindful eating can stabilize mood swings and reduce stress, which are common during menopause. By taking control of your eating patterns, you create a sense of routine and predictability, which can be incredibly grounding during a time of significant hormonal changes.

In conclusion, structuring your day around the Galveston Diet's meal timing and frequency principles can transform your approach to eating and health. By embracing intermittent fasting, focusing on balanced, nutrient-dense meals, and listening to your body's hunger signals, you can optimize your nutrition and well-being. This approach not only supports physical health but also enhances mental and emotional resilience, helping you navigate menopause with confidence and vitality. Each meal becomes an opportunity to nourish your body and honor your health, creating a harmonious rhythm that aligns with the natural cycles of your life.

INCORPORATING EXERCISE AND PHYSICAL ACTIVITY

Imagine stepping outside early in the morning, the cool breeze invigorating your senses as the first rays of sunlight break through the horizon. This peaceful moment can set the tone for incorporating exercise and physical activity into your daily routine, a key component of the Galveston Diet's approach to overall well-being.

Exercise is more than just a means to manage weight; it's a vital part of maintaining health, particularly during menopause. Regular physical activity can help mitigate some of the common symptoms of menopause, such as weight gain, mood swings, and bone density loss. It also plays a crucial role in maintaining muscle mass, improving cardiovascular health, and boosting mental clarity.

Start your day with a gentle warm-up. This could be a series of stretches or a short yoga session. Stretching not only prepares your body for more vigorous activity but also helps to improve flexibility and reduce the risk of injury. Yoga, with its focus on breath control and mindfulness, can also help to center your mind, setting a positive tone for the day ahead. Think of it as a way to greet your body, acknowledging its strength and capabilities while preparing it for the challenges ahead.

As the day progresses, find moments to integrate more substantial exercise. Perhaps you could take a brisk walk around your neighborhood or a nearby park. Walking is a low-impact exercise that's accessible to almost everyone and can be easily adjusted in intensity to match your fitness level. Walking in nature also offers the added benefit of fresh air and natural scenery, which can boost your mood and mental well-being. Research has shown that spending time outdoors can reduce stress and enhance cognitive function, making it an excellent complement to your physical fitness routine.

For those looking for a more vigorous workout, consider incorporating strength training into your schedule. Strength training is particularly beneficial during menopause as it helps to counteract the natural decline in muscle mass and bone density that occurs with age. Lifting weights, using resistance bands, or even body-weight exercises like squats and push-ups can all contribute to maintaining and building muscle strength. Aim for two to three sessions per week, focusing on different muscle groups to ensure a balanced approach.

Remember, exercise doesn't have to be confined to traditional workouts. Everyday activities like gardening, dancing, or even playing with your pets can provide significant physical benefits. The key is to stay active and find joy in movement. By viewing exercise as a part of your lifestyle rather than a chore, you're more likely to stick with it and reap the long-term benefits. Incorporating cardiovascular exercise is also crucial. Activities such as cycling, swimming, or running can improve heart health, increase lung capacity, and boost overall endurance. If you're new to these types of activities, start slowly and gradually increase your intensity and duration. For example, you might begin with a 20-minute bike ride around your neighborhood, gradually extending your ride as your fitness improves. The goal is to challenge your heart and lungs while still enjoying the activity.

One of the most powerful benefits of regular exercise is its impact on mental health. Physical activity stimulates the release of endorphins, often referred to as "feel-good" hormones, which can alleviate feelings of depression and anxiety. This is particularly relevant during menopause, a time when many women experience fluctuations in mood. Exercise provides a natural, effective way to manage stress and enhance emotional resilience.

Let's not forget the social aspect of physical activity. Joining a fitness class, a walking group, or a sports team can provide a sense of community and support. Social connections are important for emotional well-being, and exercising with others can add an element of fun and accountability. Whether it's a yoga class, a hiking club, or a dance group, sharing physical activity with others can enhance your motivation and enjoyment.

Balancing rest and recovery is equally important. Your body needs time to repair and strengthen after exercise. Ensure you get adequate sleep and consider incorporating relaxation techniques such as deep breathing exercises, meditation, or a warm bath to help your muscles recover and to promote overall relaxation. Listening to your body and giving it the rest it needs can prevent injuries and overtraining, ensuring that you can maintain a consistent exercise routine.

As evening approaches, consider a calming activity like tai chi or an evening walk. Tai chi, with its slow, deliberate movements and focus on balance and control, can be a perfect way to wind down. An evening walk can also be a peaceful end to the day, helping to signal to your body that it's time to relax and prepare for sleep.

Incorporating exercise and physical activity into your daily routine doesn't have to be complicated or time-consuming. The key is consistency and finding activities that you enjoy. By making physical activity a regular part of your day, you not only support your physical health but also enhance your mental and emotional well-being. The Galveston Diet emphasizes a holistic approach to health, and exercise is a vital component of that approach. Whether it's a morning stretch, a midday walk, or an evening tai chi session, each activity contributes to a balanced, healthy lifestyle.

In conclusion, structuring your day to include various forms of exercise can transform your approach to health during menopause. By embracing a mix of cardiovascular activities, strength training, and flexibility exercises, you create a comprehensive fitness routine that supports your body and mind. Exercise becomes more than just a means to an end; it's an integral part of a fulfilling, vibrant life. Each step, each stretch, and each movement brings you closer to a state of balance and well-being, empowering you to navigate menopause with strength and confidence.

3. Creating a Supportive Environment

Stocking Your Kitchen with Essentials

Imagine stepping into your kitchen, the heart of your home, and finding it brimming with ingredients that inspire you to create meals that nourish both your body and soul. A well-stocked kitchen is essential for embracing the Galveston Diet and ensuring you have everything you need at your fingertips to prepare healthy, delicious meals. Transforming your kitchen into a haven of health begins with understanding the essentials and how they support your journey toward hormonal balance and overall well-being during menopause.

To start, let's envision your pantry. This is your go-to place for dry goods and staples that form the foundation of many meals. Whole grains like quinoa, brown rice, and oats are excellent choices. They provide complex carbohydrates that release energy slowly, helping to keep your blood sugar levels stable and your energy steady throughout the day. Quinoa, for instance, is not only a great source of protein but also rich in fiber and essential amino acids, making it a perfect base for salads or a side dish.

Next, think about legumes and beans. Chickpeas, lentils, black beans, and kidney beans are versatile, nutrient-dense options that can be used in a variety of dishes. They are high in protein and fiber, which help keep you feeling full and satisfied. Imagine whipping up a hearty lentil soup on a chilly evening or tossing chickpeas into a salad for a protein boost. These staples are also budget-friendly and have a long shelf life, making them convenient to have on hand.

Your pantry should also include a variety of nuts and seeds. Almonds, walnuts, chia seeds, and flaxseeds are rich in healthy fats, protein, and fiber. These can be added to smoothies, sprinkled over salads, or simply enjoyed as a snack. The omega-3 fatty acids found in walnuts and flaxseeds are particularly beneficial for brain health and reducing inflammation, key concerns during menopause.

Don't forget about healthy oils and vinegars. Extra virgin olive oil is a cornerstone of the Galveston Diet, celebrated for its anti-inflammatory properties and heart-healthy benefits. Coconut oil is another good option for cooking due to its high smoke point and unique flavor. Apple cider vinegar and balsamic vinegar can enhance the flavor of your dishes and offer health benefits such as improved digestion and blood sugar control. Now, let's move to the refrigerator. This is where fresh produce, dairy, and proteins are stored.

Leafy greens like spinach, kale, and arugula should have a permanent spot on your shelves. These greens are packed with vitamins, minerals, and antioxidants that support overall health. They are incredibly versatile, perfect for salads, smoothies, or sautéed as a side dish. Think about the satisfaction of creating a colorful, nutrient-rich salad with a mix of these greens, topped with vibrant vegetables and a tangy vinaigrette.

Cruciferous vegetables like broccoli, cauliflower, and Brussels sprouts are also essential. They are known for their cancer-fighting properties and are rich in fiber and vitamins. Roasting these vegetables brings out their natural sweetness and makes them a delicious addition to any meal.

When it comes to proteins, consider lean sources like chicken, turkey, and fish. These proteins are vital for maintaining muscle mass and supporting metabolic health. Fatty fish such as salmon, mackerel, and sardines are particularly beneficial because they are high in omega-3 fatty acids. Imagine grilling a piece of salmon, seasoned simply with lemon and herbs, serving it alongside a medley of roasted vegetables for a meal that is both satisfying and packed with nutrients.

Eggs are another versatile protein source that can be used in countless ways, from breakfast omelets to lunchtime salads or dinner frittatas. They are rich in essential nutrients like choline, which supports brain health, and are relatively quick and easy to prepare.

Dairy or dairy alternatives are also important. Greek yogurt is an excellent choice because it's high in protein and probiotics, which support gut health. Use it as a base for smoothies, a topping for fruit, or a creamy addition to sauces and dressings. If you're lactose intolerant or prefer plant-based options, almond milk or oat milk are good alternatives that can be used in similar ways.

Now, let's talk about the freezer. Having a stock of frozen fruits and vegetables can be a lifesaver on busy days when fresh produce might not be available. Frozen berries, spinach, and mixed vegetables retain most of their nutrients and can be quickly added to smoothies, soups, or stir-fries. They provide a convenient and cost-effective way to ensure you're always prepared to make a healthy meal.

In addition to fruits and vegetables, consider keeping frozen fish or lean meats. These can be defrosted as needed, making meal planning more flexible. Think about how comforting it is to know you can always create a healthy, balanced meal without needing to run to the store.

Spices and herbs are the final touch to a well-stocked kitchen. These not only add flavor to your meals but also offer numerous health benefits. Turmeric, ginger, garlic, and cinnamon are powerful anti-inflammatory agents that can enhance your dishes while supporting your health. Fresh herbs like parsley, cilantro, and basil can add a burst of flavor and a dose of vitamins. Imagine the aroma of a homemade curry simmering on the stove, filled with vibrant spices and fresh herbs, creating a meal that is as healing as it is delicious.

Stocking your kitchen with these essentials creates an environment where healthy eating becomes second nature. It reduces the temptation to reach for processed or unhealthy options when you have nutritious, delicious ingredients readily available. Moreover, it sets you up for success by making meal preparation simpler and more enjoyable.

The transformation of your kitchen into a supportive environment is not just about the physical space but also about the mindset it fosters. Knowing that you have everything you need to prepare wholesome meals empowers you to make better choices and reinforces your commitment to the Galveston Diet and your health journey.

In conclusion, a well-stocked kitchen is the foundation of a successful transition to the Galveston Diet. By thoughtfully selecting and organizing your pantry, refrigerator, and freezer, you create a supportive environment that makes healthy eating effortless and enjoyable. This preparation not only supports your physical health but also nurtures a positive relationship with food, empowering you to thrive during menopause and beyond. Each ingredient you choose and each meal you prepare is a step toward a healthier, more vibrant life, guided by the principles of the Galveston Diet.

MANAGING SOCIAL SITUATIONS AND EATING OUT

Navigating social situations and eating out can be challenging when trying to maintain a healthy diet, especially one as focused and intentional as the Galveston Diet. Yet, these moments are also a vital part of our lives, providing opportunities for connection, celebration, and enjoyment. The key is to approach them with a blend of mindfulness, flexibility, and preparation, ensuring that you can enjoy these experiences without compromising your commitment to your health and well-being.

Picture yourself at a bustling restaurant, the aroma of various dishes wafting through the air. You're there to celebrate a friend's birthday, and you want to enjoy the occasion without straying from your dietary goals. The first step is to plan ahead. Many restaurants post their menus online, allowing you to review your options beforehand. Look for dishes that align with the principles of the Galveston Diet: lean proteins, plenty of vegetables, and healthy fats. This pre-planning can help reduce the stress of making decisions on the spot and ensure you have a strategy in place.

When you arrive, scan the menu with a discerning eye. Start by choosing a healthy appetizer. A salad with a light vinaigrette or a broth-based soup can be excellent choices, setting a positive tone for the rest of the meal. If you're unsure about ingredients or preparation methods, don't hesitate to ask your server. Requesting modifications, such as dressing on the side or substituting vegetables for starchy sides, is perfectly acceptable. Most restaurants are happy to accommodate dietary needs and preferences. Social situations often come with temptations, whether it's a basket of bread on the table or a dessert tray making the rounds. It's helpful to have a game plan for these moments. For instance, enjoy a piece of bread if you truly want it, but balance it by focusing on the healthier aspects of your meal. Mindfulness is your ally here. Take the time to savor each bite, appreciating the flavors and textures, which can enhance your satisfaction and prevent overeating. Drinks are another area where mindfulness plays a crucial role. Alcohol and sugary beverages can quickly add up in calories and sugar, potentially derailing your efforts. Opt for water, sparkling water with a twist of lime, or unsweetened iced tea. If you choose to have an alcoholic drink, moderation is key. A glass of wine or a simple cocktail without sugary mixers can be enjoyed responsibly. Remember, staying hydrated with water throughout the meal can also help you feel fuller and more satisfied.

Let's transition to a different scenario: a family gathering or a potluck with friends. These events often involve a variety of dishes, many of which may not align with your dietary goals. In these cases, contribution is a powerful strategy. Bring a dish or two that you know are Galveston Diet-friendly. This ensures there's at least one option that you can enjoy without reservation. Sharing healthy dishes also introduces others to the benefits of nutritious, delicious food, potentially inspiring them to make healthier choices as well.

At the buffet table, start by surveying all the options before filling your plate. This allows you to make informed choices rather than impulsively grabbing the first things you see. Aim to fill half your plate with vegetables and lean proteins, leaving smaller portions for other items. Portion control can help you enjoy a variety of foods without overindulging. Remember, it's not about depriving yourself but about making choices that support your health and well-being.

Conversations and social interactions are a big part of these gatherings. Engaging in lively discussions can naturally slow down your eating pace, giving your body time to register fullness and satisfaction. This slower pace helps you enjoy your food and the company without overeating. It's also an excellent opportunity to share your health journey with others. Talking about the Galveston Diet and its benefits can be a source of inspiration for friends and family who might be considering healthier lifestyles.

Holidays and special occasions often come with traditions and expectations around food. It's essential to find a balance that honors these traditions while still aligning with your dietary goals. For instance, if Thanksgiving is a significant celebration in your family, focus on enjoying the lean turkey and vegetable sides while being mindful of the richer, more indulgent dishes. Allow yourself to enjoy small portions of your favorite holiday treats, recognizing that these moments are part of the overall experience and can be enjoyed in moderation.

Flexibility is crucial. Life is meant to be enjoyed, and food is a significant part of that enjoyment. The Galveston Diet is not about rigid restrictions but about making informed, mindful choices that support your health. If you have a day where you indulge more than usual, approach it with kindness and understanding. The next meal is an opportunity to return to your healthier habits without guilt or regret. This balanced approach helps to maintain a positive relationship with food and reinforces that health is a long-term journey, not defined by a single meal or day.

Traveling presents another set of challenges and opportunities. When on the road, plan ahead as much as possible. Pack healthy snacks like nuts, seeds, or fruit to have on hand during long trips. Researching restaurant options in advance can also help you find places that offer healthier choices. Many cities have restaurants that cater to a variety of dietary preferences, including those that align with the Galveston Diet. Hotel breakfasts can often be a mix of healthy and indulgent options, so choose wisely. Opt for eggs, yogurt, fresh fruit, and whole-grain options rather than pastries and sugary cereals.

Ultimately, the goal is to integrate the principles of the Galveston Diet into all aspects of your life, including social situations and dining out. By planning ahead, making mindful choices, and maintaining flexibility, you can enjoy these experiences without compromising your commitment to your health. It's about creating a supportive environment that allows you to thrive, making every meal an opportunity to nourish your body and connect with others. Each social event becomes a chance to practice and reinforce your healthy habits, empowering you to maintain your well-being while fully engaging in the joys of life.

BUILDING A SUPPORT NETWORK

Imagine yourself embarking on a journey towards better health and well-being. Like any journey, it is filled with ups and downs, moments of triumph, and times of challenge. Now, imagine having a group of fellow travelers by your side, offering support, encouragement, and understanding. This is the essence of building a support network—a community that uplifts you and helps you stay committed to the Galveston Diet and your health goals.

The importance of a support network cannot be overstated. Social connections are fundamental to human nature, providing a sense of belonging and emotional security. For women navigating menopause and the lifestyle changes that come with the Galveston Diet, having a robust support system can make all the difference. Research shows that people who have strong social support are more likely to stick to their health routines, experience better mental health, and achieve their goals more effectively. Start by looking close to home. Family and friends can be a wonderful source of support.

Share your health journey with them, explaining why you've chosen the Galveston Diet and how it benefits your well-being. Open conversations can help them understand your choices and encourage them to support you. For instance, you might say, "I'm focusing on a diet that helps with inflammation and hormonal balance during menopause. It's important for my health, and I'd love your support." This invites them into your journey and helps them feel a part of it.

Having family meals together can be a great way to integrate your new dietary habits. Involve your loved ones in meal planning and preparation. Cooking together can be a fun and educational experience, allowing everyone to learn about healthy eating. Imagine preparing a vibrant salad or a delicious, lean protein dish together, chatting and laughing as you work. This not only strengthens your bond but also helps them appreciate the effort and benefits of your diet.

If your immediate family is supportive but perhaps not fully onboard with all your dietary changes, create a balance. Cook meals that align with the Galveston Diet but also include elements that they enjoy. For instance, prepare a base of roasted vegetables and lean protein, and then add sides or toppings that cater to their preferences. This way, everyone can enjoy the meal without feeling deprived, and you stay true to your health goals.

Beyond family, look to your circle of friends. Friends who share your health interests can become accountability partners. Arrange regular check-ins, whether it's a weekly coffee date or a group chat where you share your progress and challenges. Encouraging each other can keep you motivated. Picture this: meeting a friend for a brisk walk in the park, discussing your week's successes and obstacles, and feeling reinvigorated by the shared experience. These moments of connection can be incredibly reinforcing.

Online communities can also be a powerful source of support. Social media platforms, forums, and groups dedicated to the Galveston Diet or menopause wellness can connect you with like-minded individuals. These virtual spaces provide a venue to share tips, recipes, and personal stories, creating a sense of camaraderie and understanding. The anonymity of online interactions can sometimes make it easier to share openly and honestly about your experiences.

Local support groups are another excellent resource. Many communities offer groups focused on health and wellness, often through local community centers, gyms, or health clinics. Joining a group where you can meet face-to-face with others who understand your journey can be immensely rewarding. Consider attending a weekly support group meeting where you can discuss your progress, learn from guest speakers, and participate in group activities.

Professional support is equally important. Consulting with a dietitian, nutritionist, or health coach can provide you with personalized guidance and accountability. These professionals can help you tailor the Galveston Diet to your specific needs, troubleshoot any challenges, and celebrate your successes. Regular appointments with a supportive healthcare provider can give you the structure and expert advice necessary to stay on track.

Don't underestimate the power of mentorship. If you know someone who has successfully navigated menopause or adopted a similar diet, seek their guidance. A mentor can offer invaluable insights, share their experiences, and provide practical tips. This relationship can be particularly inspiring, showing you that your goals are attainable and offering a roadmap based on real-life success.

Building a support network also means giving support in return. Encourage and uplift those in your circle who are also pursuing health goals. Celebrate their successes, offer a listening ear during their challenges, and share your knowledge. This reciprocal relationship strengthens the bonds within your support network and fosters a positive, encouraging environment.

Remember, a support network is not just about others supporting you; it's also about creating an environment that supports your goals. This includes setting up your physical space—your home, your kitchen, your workspace—to align with your health objectives. Stock your kitchen with essentials that make it easy to follow the Galveston Diet, and create a schedule that prioritizes your well-being. Your environment plays a crucial role in your success, and organizing it thoughtfully can provide daily reinforcement of your commitment.

Incorporate positive affirmations and self-care practices into your routine. Surround yourself with inspirational quotes, books, and music that uplift you. Taking time for self-reflection, journaling your progress, and practicing mindfulness can enhance your emotional resilience. These personal practices complement your external support network, ensuring you are fortified from within as well.

In conclusion, building a support network is a multifaceted process that involves family, friends, online communities, local groups, and professionals. It's about creating an environment—both social and physical—that supports your health journey. By surrounding yourself with positive influences, sharing your experiences, and offering support to others, you create a strong, supportive network that helps you thrive on the Galveston Diet. This network not only aids you in reaching your health goals but also enriches your life with meaningful connections and shared experiences. Together, you can navigate the challenges and celebrate the successes, making your journey towards health and well-being a collaborative and fulfilling adventure.

4. Adapting the Lifestyle to Fit Your Needs

Customizing the Diet for Different Lifestyles

Every individual is unique, and so is their lifestyle. Whether you are a busy professional, a stay-at-home parent, or a retiree, the Galveston Diet can be tailored to fit seamlessly into your daily routine. The beauty of this diet lies in its flexibility and adaptability, allowing you to customize it according to your needs and preferences without compromising its benefits.

Let's start with the life of a busy professional. Picture a typical weekday morning: you wake up early, perhaps after a restless night, and immediately dive into the whirlwind of emails, meetings, and deadlines. It's easy to grab a quick, convenient breakfast that might not align with your health goals. Instead, with a bit of planning, you can set yourself up for success. Consider preparing a nutrient-dense breakfast the night before—perhaps overnight oats with chia seeds and berries, or a smoothie packed with greens, protein, and healthy fats. These options are quick to grab and can be enjoyed on the go, ensuring you start your day with sustained energy and focus.

Lunchtime can be equally challenging for the busy professional. You might be tempted by fast food or skip the meal altogether due to back-to-back meetings. A better approach is to prepare balanced meals in advance. Spend a bit of your weekend prepping salads with a variety of colorful vegetables, lean proteins, and a simple vinaigrette. Store them in the fridge, ready to grab as you head out the door. If you prefer a hot meal, consider batch-cooking soups or stews that can be easily reheated. By investing a little time in meal prep, you can avoid unhealthy choices and fuel your body with the nutrients it needs to power through the day.

Now imagine the lifestyle of a stay-at-home parent. Your days are filled with taking care of your family, managing the household, and juggling countless responsibilities. Amidst the chaos, it's crucial to prioritize your own health. Involve your family in meal planning and preparation. This not only lightens your load but also teaches children about healthy eating habits. You could designate a day for everyone to cook together, making it a fun and educational activity. For instance, preparing a colorful vegetable stir-fry with lean protein can become a family event, where each member adds their favorite veggies to the mix. This way, you ensure that everyone's tastes are considered, and you reinforce the importance of healthy eating.

Snacking can be a pitfall when you're constantly on the move at home. Instead of reaching for processed snacks, stock your pantry with healthy options like nuts, seeds, and fresh fruit. Pre-portioning these snacks can help you manage your intake and avoid mindless eating. Additionally, keeping a bowl of washed and cut vegetables in the fridge makes it easy to grab a healthy snack when you need a quick bite. For retirees, the transition to a slower pace of life offers a wonderful opportunity to focus on health and well-being.

With more time on your hands, you can explore new recipes and cooking techniques that align with the Galveston Diet. Visit local farmers' markets to find fresh, seasonal produce, and experiment with different ways to prepare and enjoy these foods. Cooking can become a relaxing and rewarding hobby, one that not only benefits your health but also brings joy and satisfaction.

Staying active is another important aspect of the Galveston Diet for retirees. Incorporating regular physical activity into your routine can enhance the benefits of the diet and improve overall well-being. Whether it's taking a daily walk, joining a local fitness class, or practicing yoga, staying active helps maintain muscle mass, supports cardiovascular health, and boosts mood. Pairing these activities with a balanced diet ensures that you're nurturing your body and mind in harmony.

For those with dietary restrictions or preferences, the Galveston Diet is versatile enough to accommodate. If you're vegetarian or vegan, focus on plant-based proteins like legumes, tofu, and tempeh. These can be combined with a variety of vegetables and whole grains to create satisfying and nutritious meals. If you're gluten-free, there are plenty of alternatives such as quinoa, rice, and gluten-free oats that fit perfectly into the diet. The key is to focus on whole, unprocessed foods that provide the nutrients your body needs.

Travel can also pose a challenge, but with a little planning, you can stay on track with the Galveston Diet. When traveling, pack healthy snacks such as nuts, seeds, and dried fruit to avoid the temptation of airport food or convenience store options. Research restaurants at your destination that offer healthy choices, and don't hesitate to ask for modifications to suit your dietary needs. Staying hydrated is crucial, so carry a water bottle and sip regularly, especially during flights. By being mindful and prepared, you can enjoy your travels without compromising your health goals.

Social gatherings and dining out are part of life's pleasures, and they don't have to derail your dietary efforts. When dining out, choose restaurants that offer healthy options and don't be afraid to ask for modifications. Opt for dishes that include plenty of vegetables, lean proteins, and healthy fats. If you're attending a social gathering, offer to bring a dish that aligns with your dietary preferences. This ensures there's something you can enjoy while also sharing the benefits of healthy eating with others.

Flexibility and balance are at the heart of customizing the Galveston Diet for different lifestyles. It's about finding what works best for you, making adjustments as needed, and embracing a mindful approach to eating. Life is dynamic, and your diet should be adaptable to fit your unique circumstances. By focusing on whole, nutrient-dense foods and listening to your body's needs, you can thrive on the Galveston Diet, no matter your lifestyle.

In conclusion, the Galveston Diet's adaptability makes it an ideal choice for a variety of lifestyles. Whether you're a busy professional, a stay-at-home parent, a retiree, or someone with specific dietary needs, the diet can be tailored to support your health goals. By planning ahead, staying mindful, and embracing flexibility, you can integrate the principles of the Galveston Diet into your daily routine, ensuring that you nourish your body and mind effectively. This personalized approach not only enhances your physical health but also enriches your overall quality of life, empowering you to live fully and vibrantly.

CHAPTER 2: MINDSET AND GOALS

1. Setting Realistic and Achievable Goals

Defining Your Personal Objectives

Every individual is unique, and so is their lifestyle. Whether you are a busy professional, a stay-at-home parent, or a retiree, the Galveston Diet can be tailored to fit seamlessly into your daily routine. The beauty of this diet lies in its flexibility and adaptability, allowing you to customize it according to your needs and preferences without compromising its benefits.

Let's start with the life of a busy professional. Picture a typical weekday morning: you wake up early, perhaps after a restless night, and immediately dive into the whirlwind of emails, meetings, and deadlines. It's easy to grab a quick, convenient breakfast that might not align with your health goals. Instead, with a bit of planning, you can set yourself up for success. Consider preparing a nutrient-dense breakfast the night before—perhaps overnight oats with chia seeds and berries, or a smoothie packed with greens, protein, and healthy fats. These options are quick to grab and can be enjoyed on the go, ensuring you start your day with sustained energy and focus.

Lunchtime can be equally challenging for the busy professional. You might be tempted by fast food or skip the meal altogether due to back-to-back meetings. A better approach is to prepare balanced meals in advance. Spend a bit of your weekend prepping salads with a variety of colorful vegetables, lean proteins, and a simple vinaigrette. Store them in the fridge, ready to grab as you head out the door. If you prefer a hot meal, consider batch-cooking soups or stews that can be easily reheated. By investing a little time in meal prep, you can avoid unhealthy choices and fuel your body with the nutrients it needs to power through the day.

Now imagine the lifestyle of a stay-at-home parent. Your days are filled with taking care of your family, managing the household, and juggling countless responsibilities. Amidst the chaos, it's crucial to prioritize your own health. Involve your family in meal planning and preparation. This not only lightens your load but also teaches children about healthy eating habits. You could designate a day for everyone to cook together, making it a fun and educational activity. For instance, preparing a colorful vegetable stir-fry with lean protein can become a family event, where each member adds their favorite veggies to the mix. This way, you ensure that everyone's tastes are considered, and you reinforce the importance of healthy eating.

Snacking can be a pitfall when you're constantly on the move at home. Instead of reaching for processed snacks, stock your pantry with healthy options like nuts, seeds, and fresh fruit. Pre-portioning these snacks can help you manage your intake and avoid mindless eating. Additionally, keeping a bowl of washed and cut vegetables in the fridge makes it easy to grab a healthy snack when you need a quick bite.

For retirees, the transition to a slower pace of life offers a wonderful opportunity to focus on health and well-being. With more time on your hands, you can explore new recipes and cooking techniques that align with the Galveston Diet. Visit local farmers' markets to find fresh, seasonal produce, and experiment with different ways to prepare and enjoy these foods. Cooking can become a relaxing and rewarding hobby, one that not only benefits your health but also brings joy and satisfaction.

Staying active is another important aspect of the Galveston Diet for retirees. Incorporating regular physical activity into your routine can enhance the benefits of the diet and improve overall well-being. Whether it's taking a daily walk, joining a local fitness class, or practicing yoga, staying active helps maintain muscle mass, supports cardiovascular health, and boosts mood. Pairing these activities with a balanced diet ensures that you're nurturing your body and mind in harmony. For those with dietary restrictions or preferences, the Galveston Diet is versatile enough to accommodate. If you're vegetarian or vegan, focus on plant-based proteins like legumes, tofu, and tempeh. These can be combined with a variety of vegetables and whole grains to create satisfying and nutritious meals. If you're gluten-free, there are plenty of alternatives such as quinoa, rice, and gluten-free oats that fit perfectly into the diet. The key is to focus on whole, unprocessed foods that provide the nutrients your body needs.

Travel can also pose a challenge, but with a little planning, you can stay on track with the Galveston Diet. When traveling, pack healthy snacks such as nuts, seeds, and dried fruit to avoid the temptation of airport food or convenience store options. Research restaurants at your destination that offer healthy choices, and don't hesitate to ask for modifications to suit your dietary needs. Staying hydrated is crucial, so carry a water bottle and sip regularly, especially during flights. By being mindful and prepared, you can enjoy your travels without compromising your health goals. Social gatherings and dining out are part of life's pleasures, and they don't have to derail your dietary efforts. When dining out, choose restaurants that offer healthy options and don't be afraid to ask for modifications. Opt for dishes that include plenty of vegetables, lean proteins, and healthy fats. If you're attending a social gathering, offer to bring a dish that aligns with your dietary preferences. This ensures there's something you can enjoy while also sharing the benefits of healthy eating with others.

Flexibility and balance are at the heart of customizing the Galveston Diet for different lifestyles. It's about finding what works best for you, making adjustments as needed, and embracing a mindful approach to eating. Life is dynamic, and your diet should be adaptable to fit your unique circumstances. By focusing on whole, nutrient-dense foods and listening to your body's needs, you can thrive on the Galveston Diet, no matter your lifestyle.

In conclusion, the Galveston Diet's adaptability makes it an ideal choice for a variety of lifestyles. Whether you're a busy professional, a stay-at-home parent, a retiree, or someone with specific dietary needs, the diet can be tailored to support your health goals. By planning ahead, staying mindful, and embracing flexibility, you can integrate the principles of the Galveston Diet into your daily routine, ensuring that you nourish your body and mind effectively. This personalized approach not only enhances your physical health but also enriches your overall quality of life, empowering you to live fully and vibrantly.

SHORT-TERM VS. LONG-TERM GOALS

Setting goals is a vital part of any journey, especially one that involves transforming your health and lifestyle through the Galveston Diet. Understanding the distinction between short-term and long-term goals is crucial for staying motivated and achieving lasting success. Both types of goals serve unique purposes and, when used together, create a comprehensive roadmap to guide you on your path to better health.

Short-term goals are the stepping stones that pave the way to long-term success. They are immediate, actionable, and often focus on the smaller, day-to-day changes that build up to larger achievements. Think of short-term goals as the quick wins that keep you motivated and moving forward. For example, a short-term goal might be to incorporate more vegetables into your daily meals or to drink a certain amount of water each day. These goals are specific, measurable, and attainable within a short period, making them easier to track and achieve.

Imagine waking up on a Monday morning, feeling determined to start the week on a healthy note. You set a short-term goal to prepare a nutritious breakfast each day, something simple and achievable like a smoothie packed with greens, berries, and a scoop of protein powder. Each morning, as you blend your ingredients and enjoy your smoothie, you experience the immediate satisfaction of making a healthy choice. This daily success reinforces your commitment to the Galveston Diet and builds a positive momentum that can carry you through the week.

Short-term goals also provide opportunities to celebrate progress. These small victories are crucial for maintaining motivation, especially when the journey feels challenging. Celebrating these wins can be as simple as acknowledging your success at the end of each day or week, or treating yourself to a non-food reward, such as a relaxing bath or a new book. Recognizing and celebrating these achievements helps to build a positive mindset and encourages continued effort.

While short-term goals focus on immediate actions, long-term goals are the broader, overarching objectives that reflect your ultimate vision for health and well-being. These goals often require sustained effort and a longer timeframe to achieve, but they provide a sense of direction and purpose. A long-term goal might be to reach a healthy weight, improve your cholesterol levels, or enhance your overall energy and vitality. These goals represent the end results of your commitment to the Galveston Diet and lifestyle changes.

Visualizing your long-term goals can be a powerful motivator. Picture yourself a year from now, feeling vibrant and full of energy. You've reached your target weight, your lab results are excellent, and you feel more confident in your body. This vision serves as a constant reminder of why you embarked on this journey in the first place. It helps to keep you focused during challenging times and provides a benchmark against which you can measure your progress.

One effective strategy for staying on track with long-term goals is to break them down into smaller, manageable steps. This is where short-term goals come into play. By aligning your short-term actions with your long-term objectives, you create a clear pathway to success. For instance, if your long-term goal is to lower your cholesterol levels, a series of short-term goals could include incorporating more fiber-rich foods into your diet, reducing your intake of saturated fats, and increasing your physical activity. Each of these smaller goals contributes to the larger objective, making the overall process more manageable and less overwhelming.

Another key aspect of setting realistic and achievable goals is flexibility. Life is unpredictable, and there will be times when you face setbacks or obstacles. It's important to approach your goals with a mindset of adaptability. If you encounter a challenge, such as a busy week at work or a family event, adjust your short-term goals to fit the circumstances. Perhaps you can't prepare a full meal every night, but you can still choose healthier options when dining out or snack on nutritious foods. Flexibility allows you to stay committed to your long-term goals without feeling defeated by temporary setbacks.

Support is also essential in achieving both short-term and long-term goals. Sharing your goals with family, friends, or a supportive community can provide accountability and encouragement. When others know about your objectives, they can offer support, celebrate your successes, and help you stay motivated during difficult times. Consider finding a workout buddy, joining an online health community, or seeking guidance from a health coach. These connections can make a significant difference in your journey.

Tracking your progress is another effective way to stay motivated and ensure you're on the right path. Keep a journal or use a digital app to log your daily actions and reflect on your progress. Note how your body feels, any changes in your energy levels, and your overall mood. Regularly reviewing your progress helps to identify patterns, celebrate milestones, and adjust your goals as needed. This ongoing reflection reinforces your commitment and allows you to make informed decisions about your health.

Lastly, it's important to maintain a positive and compassionate attitude towards yourself. Change is a gradual process, and it's normal to experience ups and downs. Celebrate your efforts and achievements, no matter how small they may seem. If you encounter setbacks, view them as learning opportunities rather than failures. Remind yourself of the progress you've made and the reasons why you embarked on this journey. A positive mindset fosters resilience and keeps you focused on your long-term vision.

In conclusion, setting realistic and achievable goals involves a balance of short-term and long-term objectives. Short-term goals provide immediate motivation and opportunities for celebration, while long-term goals offer direction and purpose. By aligning these goals, maintaining flexibility, seeking support, tracking your progress, and cultivating a positive mindset, you create a sustainable path to success with the Galveston Diet. This approach not only enhances your physical health but also empowers you to live a vibrant and fulfilling life. Each goal, whether small or large, brings you closer to your vision of optimal health and well-being.

MEASURING SUCCESS AND PROGRESS

Imagine setting out on a journey without a map or a compass. How would you know if you were heading in the right direction or making any progress at all? Measuring success and progress is like having that map and compass; it helps you stay on course, reassures you that you're making strides, and guides you when adjustments are needed. On the Galveston Diet, understanding how to measure your success and track your progress is crucial for maintaining motivation and achieving your health goals.

Success on the Galveston Diet is multifaceted, encompassing physical health, emotional well-being, and overall quality of life. To begin, it's important to recognize that success looks different for everyone. For some, it might mean losing a certain amount of weight or reducing inflammation. For others, it might be about gaining more energy, improving mood, or experiencing fewer menopausal symptoms. Defining what success means to you is the first step in measuring it effectively.

Start with setting clear, specific, and realistic goals. Instead of vague objectives like "get healthier," pinpoint measurable outcomes such as "lose 10 pounds in three months" or "reduce hot flashes by half." These specific goals give you a concrete target to aim for and make it easier to track your progress.

One of the most straightforward ways to measure progress is through regular check-ins with your weight and body measurements. However, it's crucial to remember that the scale is just one tool and doesn't tell the whole story.

For many women, especially during menopause, weight can fluctuate due to hormonal changes, water retention, and other factors. Therefore, complementing weight measurements with other metrics can provide a more comprehensive picture.

Consider keeping track of your body measurements—waist, hips, thighs, and arms—once a month. These measurements can often reveal changes that the scale doesn't, such as inches lost or muscle gained. Taking progress photos can also be incredibly motivating. Sometimes the visual evidence of your transformation is more impactful than numbers on a scale or tape measure.

Health markers are another critical aspect of measuring success. Regular check-ups with your healthcare provider can help monitor important indicators like blood pressure, cholesterol levels, blood sugar levels, and markers of inflammation. Improvements in these areas are often a direct result of dietary changes and can be more significant than weight loss alone. For example, lowering your cholesterol levels or stabilizing blood sugar can drastically reduce your risk of chronic diseases and improve your overall health.

Tracking your energy levels and mood is equally important. Many women on the Galveston Diet report increased energy and better mood regulation as they progress. Keeping a daily journal where you note your energy levels, mood, sleep quality, and any menopausal symptoms can help you see patterns and improvements over time. Reflecting on these notes periodically allows you to recognize progress that might not be immediately visible but has a profound impact on your quality of life.

Dietary adherence and habits are also key metrics. Using a food journal to log what you eat can be very insightful. It not only helps you stay accountable but also allows you to identify any foods that might trigger negative symptoms or inflammation. Over time, you'll see patterns in your eating habits, making it easier to make adjustments that align with your health goals. For example, if you notice that certain foods consistently lead to digestive issues or energy slumps, you can tweak your diet to avoid them.

Exercise is another area where progress should be measured. Whether you're walking, doing yoga, or lifting weights, tracking your physical activity helps you stay committed and see improvements in strength, endurance, and flexibility. Keep a log of your workouts, noting the duration, intensity, and any personal records or milestones. This not only helps you stay motivated but also ensures that you're incorporating a balanced mix of activities that support overall health.

Let's not overlook the importance of mental and emotional well-being. Stress reduction, improved self-esteem, and better coping mechanisms are all signs of success on the Galveston Diet. Mindfulness practices, such as meditation or deep breathing exercises, can be tracked through journaling or apps that monitor your progress.

These practices contribute significantly to overall health and can enhance your dietary efforts by reducing stress-related eating and improving emotional resilience.

Social support and engagement are also indicators of progress. Building a support network and engaging with others on a similar journey can provide encouragement, accountability, and shared experiences. Participating in support groups, either in person or online, and attending community events related to health and wellness can enrich your journey and offer a sense of belonging and motivation.

Finally, celebrate your successes, no matter how small. Each milestone—whether it's a pound lost, a healthy meal prepared, or a new fitness goal achieved—deserves recognition. Celebrating these wins helps reinforce positive behavior and keeps you motivated. Rewards don't have to be extravagant; they can be as simple as treating yourself to a relaxing activity, a new book, or a day out with friends.

In conclusion, measuring success and progress on the Galveston Diet involves a holistic approach that includes physical, emotional, and social dimensions. By setting specific, realistic goals and using a variety of metrics to track your journey, you can gain a comprehensive understanding of your progress. Regular check-ins, journaling, and reflecting on your journey help to keep you motivated and ensure that you're moving in the right direction. Remember, success is not just about the destination but also about the positive changes and growth experienced along the way. Each step you take brings you closer to a healthier, more vibrant you, and that in itself is a significant achievement.

2. Cultivating a Positive Mindset

Overcoming Negative Self-Talk

Imagine standing in front of the mirror, examining your reflection with a critical eye. Your mind begins to whisper thoughts of doubt and self-criticism. "I'm not doing enough." "I'll never reach my goals." These thoughts are all too familiar to many of us, yet they can be the biggest obstacles on our journey to health and well-being. Overcoming negative self-talk is crucial for cultivating a positive mindset, especially when adopting a new lifestyle like the Galveston Diet.

Negative self-talk can be insidious, often creeping in during moments of vulnerability or stress. It's important to recognize that these thoughts are not truths but rather reflections of our fears and insecurities. The first step in overcoming negative self-talk is to become aware of it. Start by paying attention to your inner dialogue. When you catch yourself thinking something negative, pause and take note. This awareness is the foundation for change.

Let's explore the story of Lisa, a woman who embarked on the Galveston Diet with high hopes. Initially, Lisa was excited and motivated, but as the weeks passed, she began to struggle with self-doubt. Whenever she slipped from her dietary goals, she would berate herself with thoughts like, "I've failed again" or "I'm not strong enough." These thoughts sapped her motivation and made her feel defeated.

Lisa decided to tackle her negative self-talk head-on. She began by journaling her thoughts, noting whenever she had a negative reaction to herself or her progress. This exercise helped her see patterns in her thinking. She realized that she was often hardest on herself during stressful times at work or after social gatherings where she felt pressured to eat differently.

One powerful technique Lisa used was reframing her thoughts. Instead of thinking, "I've failed again," she learned to say, "I've faced a challenge, and I'm learning from it." This shift in perspective helped her see setbacks as opportunities for growth rather than failures. Reframing is about turning negative statements into neutral or positive ones, thereby changing the narrative you tell yourself.

Another strategy Lisa employed was practicing self-compassion. She started treating herself with the same kindness and understanding that she would offer a friend. When she encountered a setback, she reminded herself that everyone makes mistakes and that she was on a journey of learning and self-improvement. This approach helped her build resilience and maintain her motivation.

Lisa also found it helpful to surround herself with positive affirmations. She wrote encouraging statements and placed them around her home—in the bathroom, on the refrigerator, and even in her car.

Phrases like "I am capable," "I am making progress," and "I deserve to be healthy" became her daily mantras. These affirmations helped counteract the negative thoughts that had previously dominated her mind.

Visualization was another tool Lisa used to overcome negative self-talk. Each morning, she took a few minutes to visualize her success. She imagined herself feeling vibrant and healthy, enjoying nutritious meals, and being active. This practice not only motivated her but also reinforced her belief in her ability to achieve her goals. Visualization creates a mental image of success, making it feel more attainable and real.

Mindfulness and meditation played significant roles in Lisa's journey. By practicing mindfulness, she learned to stay present and not dwell on past mistakes or future anxieties. Meditation helped her calm her mind, reduce stress, and create a positive inner environment. Even just a few minutes of deep breathing and mindfulness each day can make a significant difference in how we perceive ourselves and our challenges.

Building a support network was crucial for Lisa. She joined an online community of women following the Galveston Diet, where she could share her experiences and receive encouragement. This sense of community provided her with the understanding and support she needed. Sharing her journey with others who were facing similar challenges made her feel less alone and more empowered.

Positive self-talk and overcoming negativity is not a one-time effort but an ongoing practice. There will be days when negative thoughts resurface, but having strategies in place can help manage them. Lisa found that regular reflection and adjustment were key. She set aside time each week to review her progress, acknowledge her achievements, and plan for the week ahead. This routine helped her stay focused and positive.

Another critical aspect is gratitude. Lisa began keeping a gratitude journal, noting things she was thankful for each day. This practice shifted her focus from what was lacking to what was abundant in her life. Gratitude helps create a positive mindset by highlighting the good, even in small everyday moments.

Exercise also became an ally in Lisa's fight against negative self-talk. Physical activity releases endorphins, the body's natural mood lifters. Lisa discovered that when she felt strong physically, she also felt more empowered mentally. Whether it was a brisk walk, a yoga session, or a dance class, moving her body helped her shake off negativity and embrace a more positive outlook.

In conclusion, overcoming negative self-talk is a vital component of cultivating a positive mindset. It requires awareness, reframing thoughts, practicing self-compassion, and employing various techniques like visualization, mindfulness, and building a support network.

Each person's journey is unique, but the principles remain the same. By consistently applying these strategies, you can transform your inner dialogue, bolster your confidence, and stay motivated on your path to health and well-being with the Galveston Diet. Remember, every step forward, no matter how small, is a victory worth celebrating.

DEVELOPING RESILIENCE AND PATIENCE

Resilience and patience are essential qualities for navigating life's challenges, particularly when adopting a new lifestyle like the Galveston Diet. These attributes enable us to stay committed to our goals, bounce back from setbacks, and maintain a positive mindset even when progress seems slow. Developing resilience and patience is a journey, but with intentional practice, you can strengthen these traits and apply them to your health and wellness journey.

Resilience begins with the ability to adapt to change and recover from difficulties. Picture yourself in the midst of a busy week, juggling work, family, and personal responsibilities. You might encounter unexpected obstacles—perhaps a sudden deadline at work or a family member falling ill. These disruptions can throw off your routine, making it challenging to stick to your dietary goals. Resilience is what allows you to adapt and continue moving forward despite these challenges.

Consider the story of Jane, a woman who embraced the Galveston Diet to improve her health during menopause. Jane faced numerous obstacles, from social pressures at family gatherings to unexpected travel for work. Each time she encountered a challenge, she reminded herself of her long-term goals and adjusted her approach. When traveling, she researched restaurants in advance to find healthy options and packed snacks that aligned with her diet. At family events, she brought her own dishes to share, ensuring she had something nutritious to eat.

Jane's resilience was bolstered by her ability to remain flexible and resourceful. She understood that perfection was not the goal; rather, it was about making the best choices possible in each situation. By viewing challenges as opportunities to learn and grow, Jane cultivated a mindset that enabled her to stay committed to her health journey.

Developing resilience also involves cultivating a strong support network. Surrounding yourself with positive influences—friends, family, or online communities—provides encouragement and perspective. When Jane felt overwhelmed, she reached out to her support network for advice and motivation. Sharing her struggles and triumphs with others who understood her journey helped her feel less isolated and more empowered.

Patience, the twin sister of resilience, is equally important. It's the ability to endure delays and setbacks without becoming discouraged.

In a world that often values instant gratification, patience can be a challenging trait to develop. However, the rewards of cultivating patience are immense, especially when it comes to long-term health goals.

Let's take a closer look at patience through the lens of Sam's experience. Sam started the Galveston Diet with the expectation of quick results. When the scale didn't immediately reflect his efforts, he felt frustrated and demotivated. Over time, Sam learned to shift his focus from immediate outcomes to the broader picture. He started celebrating non-scale victories, such as improved energy levels, better sleep, and reduced menopausal symptoms.

By recognizing and appreciating these smaller milestones, Sam developed a greater sense of patience. He understood that lasting change takes time and that each step forward, no matter how small, was progress. Patience allowed Sam to stay committed to his goals without being derailed by temporary setbacks.

Mindfulness practices can significantly enhance both resilience and patience. Techniques such as meditation, deep breathing, and mindful eating help you stay present and grounded. When you focus on the present moment, you're less likely to be overwhelmed by future anxieties or past regrets. Mindfulness teaches you to accept each moment as it is, fostering a sense of calm and patience.

For instance, when Sam felt impatient about his progress, he practiced mindful eating. He paid close attention to the flavors, textures, and aromas of his food, savoring each bite without distraction. This practice not only improved his relationship with food but also helped him appreciate the effort he was putting into his health journey.

Another key aspect of developing resilience and patience is setting realistic expectations. Understand that setbacks are a natural part of any journey, and perfection is neither achievable nor necessary. By setting achievable goals and allowing yourself grace when things don't go as planned, you build a foundation for sustained progress.

Consider keeping a journal to reflect on your journey. Documenting your thoughts, challenges, and achievements can provide valuable insights and reinforce your commitment. When you encounter a setback, write about what happened, how it made you feel, and what you learned from the experience. This reflective practice helps you process emotions and develop strategies for future challenges.

Positive self-talk is another powerful tool for building resilience and patience. Replace negative, self-critical thoughts with affirmations that reinforce your capabilities and worth. Instead of saying, "I can't do this," tell yourself, "I am capable and committed to my health." These affirmations help to rewire your brain, fostering a more positive and resilient mindset.

Engaging in regular physical activity also plays a role in developing these qualities. Exercise releases endorphins, the body's natural stress relievers, which can improve your mood and resilience. Additionally, physical activity teaches you discipline and patience as you work towards fitness goals. Whether it's yoga, walking, or strength training, find an activity you enjoy and make it a regular part of your routine.

Lastly, remember to celebrate your progress. Each step forward, no matter how small, is an achievement worth recognizing. Celebrating your successes reinforces your commitment and boosts your motivation. Treat yourself to something special, whether it's a relaxing spa day, a new book, or simply taking time to enjoy a favorite hobby.

In conclusion, developing resilience and patience is essential for cultivating a positive mindset and achieving long-term health goals. By embracing flexibility, building a support network, practicing mindfulness, setting realistic expectations, engaging in positive self-talk, and celebrating your progress, you can strengthen these traits. Resilience and patience will not only help you navigate the challenges of the Galveston Diet but also enrich your overall well-being. Remember, the journey to health is a marathon, not a sprint. With resilience and patience, you can stay the course and achieve your goals, one step at a time.

TECHNIQUES FOR STAYING MOTIVATED

Staying motivated on any health journey can be challenging, especially when adopting a new lifestyle like the Galveston Diet. Maintaining enthusiasm and commitment over the long term requires more than just initial determination; it involves a strategic approach that includes setting clear goals, finding inspiration, and cultivating a supportive environment. Let's explore techniques to stay motivated, drawing from real-life experiences and practical advice to help you keep moving forward.

Think of motivation as a fire that needs constant tending. At the start, the excitement of a new diet or lifestyle change fuels the flames, but as the novelty wears off, the fire can begin to dim. This is where setting clear, specific goals becomes crucial. Instead of vague resolutions like "eat healthier" or "lose weight," set concrete, measurable objectives. For example, aim to incorporate at least five servings of vegetables into your daily meals or walk 10,000 steps each day. These specific targets give you a clear direction and provide tangible benchmarks to celebrate along the way.

Imagine the journey of Sarah, a woman who started the Galveston Diet with the goal of improving her energy levels and reducing menopausal symptoms. Sarah found that breaking her long-term goals into smaller, short-term milestones helped her stay motivated. She set weekly objectives, such as trying a new vegetable recipe or increasing her daily water intake.

Each small success gave her a sense of accomplishment and kept her motivated to continue. Tracking your progress is another powerful way to stay motivated. Keep a journal or use a digital app to log your daily meals, exercise, and how you feel. Reviewing your entries can provide valuable insights into what works best for you and highlight the progress you've made, even if the changes seem small. This practice not only reinforces your commitment but also serves as a reminder of how far you've come. When Sarah felt her motivation waning, she looked back at her journal and saw the positive changes she had achieved, which reinvigorated her determination.

Visual reminders can also play a significant role in maintaining motivation. Create a vision board with images and quotes that represent your health goals and the vibrant life you envision for yourself. Place it somewhere you'll see it daily, such as your kitchen or bathroom mirror. These visual cues can reignite your passion and keep your goals at the forefront of your mind. For Sarah, seeing pictures of nutritious meals, active women, and serene nature scenes reminded her of the healthy, balanced life she was striving for.

Finding inspiration in others can be incredibly motivating. Join online communities or local groups where you can share your journey, ask questions, and celebrate successes with like-minded individuals. Hearing stories of others who have successfully navigated similar challenges can provide encouragement and practical tips. Sarah joined an online support group for women following the Galveston Diet, where she found camaraderie and inspiration. The shared experiences and advice from the group helped her feel supported and motivated.

Accountability partners can be invaluable. Whether it's a friend, family member, or colleague, having someone to share your goals with and report your progress to can keep you on track. Arrange regular check-ins, whether it's a weekly phone call, a shared meal prep session, or a workout together. This accountability creates a sense of responsibility and encourages you to stay committed. Sarah partnered with a coworker who also wanted to improve her health. They supported each other through lunchtime walks and shared healthy recipes, which kept both of them motivated.

Incorporating variety into your routine can prevent boredom and keep your motivation high. Experiment with new recipes, try different types of exercise, and explore various relaxation techniques. This variety not only keeps things interesting but also helps you discover what you enjoy most. For instance, Sarah tried yoga, swimming, and hiking, finding that each activity brought unique benefits and joy. This exploration helped her maintain enthusiasm for her fitness routine.

Mindfulness and positive thinking are essential components of staying motivated. Practice mindfulness by focusing on the present moment and appreciating the small victories each day brings. This could be as simple as savoring the taste of a healthy meal or enjoying the feeling of a good workout. Positive thinking involves reframing challenges as opportunities and setbacks as learning experiences. When Sarah faced a tough day, she reminded herself of the progress she had made and viewed the challenge as a chance to grow stronger.

Self-compassion is also crucial. Be kind to yourself and recognize that setbacks are a natural part of any journey. Instead of being overly critical, treat yourself with the same kindness and understanding you would offer a friend. If you miss a workout or indulge in an unhealthy meal, acknowledge it without judgment and refocus on your goals. This approach helps prevent the all-or-nothing mentality that can derail your progress. Sarah learned to forgive herself for occasional slip-ups and used them as motivation to continue her efforts.

Celebrating milestones is a powerful motivator. Recognize and reward yourself for achieving your goals, no matter how small they may seem. These rewards don't have to be extravagant; they could be a relaxing bath, a new book, or a night out with friends. Celebrations reinforce your achievements and provide a sense of satisfaction and encouragement to keep going. When Sarah reached her monthly fitness goals, she treated herself to a massage or a new piece of workout gear, which kept her motivated and happy.

Incorporating gratitude into your daily routine can also boost motivation. Take a few moments each day to reflect on what you're grateful for, whether it's your health, your support network, or the small victories you've achieved. Gratitude shifts your focus from what's lacking to what's abundant, fostering a positive outlook that fuels motivation. Sarah kept a gratitude journal, noting down three things she was thankful for each evening. This practice helped her end each day on a positive note and stay motivated.

Lastly, remember that motivation ebbs and flows. It's natural to have periods of high motivation and times when it feels more challenging to stay committed. During those low periods, reconnect with your reasons for starting the journey and lean on your support network. By implementing these techniques, you can build a resilient mindset that keeps you motivated, even when the going gets tough.

In conclusion, staying motivated on the Galveston Diet involves setting clear goals, tracking progress, finding inspiration, and cultivating a supportive environment. By using techniques such as visualization, mindfulness, self-compassion, and celebrating milestones, you can maintain your motivation and achieve lasting success. Remember, motivation is not a constant state but a journey. Embrace it with patience and persistence, and you will find the strength to reach your health and wellness goals.

CHAPTER 3: BREAKFASTS

AVOCADO AND SMOKED SALMON BREAKFAST BOWL

PREPARATION TIME: 10 min.
COOKING TIME: 0 min.
MODE OF COOKING: Assembling
INGREDIENTS:
- 1 ripe avocado, diced
- 4 oz smoked salmon, sliced
- 1 cup mixed greens
- 1/2 cup cherry tomatoes, halved
- 2 Tbsp red onion, finely chopped
- 2 Tbsp capers
- 2 hard-boiled eggs, quartered
- Juice of 1/2 lemon
- 1 Tbsp olive oil
- Salt and pepper to taste

DIRECTIONS:
1. In a medium bowl, combine mixed greens, cherry tomatoes, red onion, and capers.
2. Arrange diced avocado and smoked salmon on top of the salad mixture.
3. Add the quartered hard-boiled eggs around the bowl.
4. Drizzle with lemon juice and olive oil.
5. Season with salt and pepper to taste.

TIPS:
- Serve with whole-grain toast for added fiber.
- Sprinkle with fresh dill for extra flavor.

NUTRITIONAL VALUES: Calories: 380, Fat: 28g, Carbs: 12g, Protein: 22g, Sugar: 2g

SPINACH AND MUSHROOM FRITTATA

PREPARATION TIME: 10 min.
COOKING TIME: 20 min.
MODE OF COOKING: Baking
INGREDIENTS:
- 6 large eggs
- 1/2 cup unsweetened almond milk
- 1 cup fresh spinach, chopped
- 1/2 cup mushrooms, sliced
- 1/4 cup onion, diced
- 1/4 cup feta cheese, crumbled
- 1 Tbsp olive oil
- Salt and pepper to taste

DIRECTIONS:
1. Preheat oven to 375°F (190°C).
2. In a large bowl, whisk together eggs and almond milk. Season with salt and pepper.
3. Heat olive oil in an oven-safe skillet over medium heat. Add onion and mushrooms, sauté until soft.
4. Add spinach to the skillet and cook until wilted.
5. Pour the egg mixture over the vegetables and cook until the edges begin to set.
6. Sprinkle feta cheese on top and transfer the skillet to the oven.
7. Bake for 10-15 minutes, until the

frittata is fully set and slightly golden on top.

TIPS:
- Add a pinch of nutmeg to the egg mixture for a hint of warmth.
- Serve with a side of fresh fruit for a complete meal.

NUTRITIONAL VALUES: Calories: 200, Fat: 15g, Carbs: 5g, Protein: 13g, Sugar: 2g

GREEK YOGURT PARFAIT WITH BERRIES AND NUTS

PREPARATION TIME: 5 min.
COOKING TIME: 0 min.
MODE OF COOKING: Assembling
INGREDIENTS:
- 2 cups plain Greek yogurt
- 1/2 cup mixed berries (blueberries, strawberries, raspberries)
- 1/4 cup granola (low-sugar)
- 2 Tbsp chopped nuts (almonds, walnuts)
- 1 Tbsp honey

DIRECTIONS:
1. In two serving glasses, layer Greek yogurt, mixed berries, granola, and nuts.
2. Drizzle honey on top.
3. Serve immediately.

TIPS:
- Use fresh or frozen berries based on availability.
- Add a sprinkle of cinnamon for extra flavor.

NUTRITIONAL VALUES: Calories: 250, Fat: 9g, Carbs: 28g, Protein: 17g, Sugar: 16g

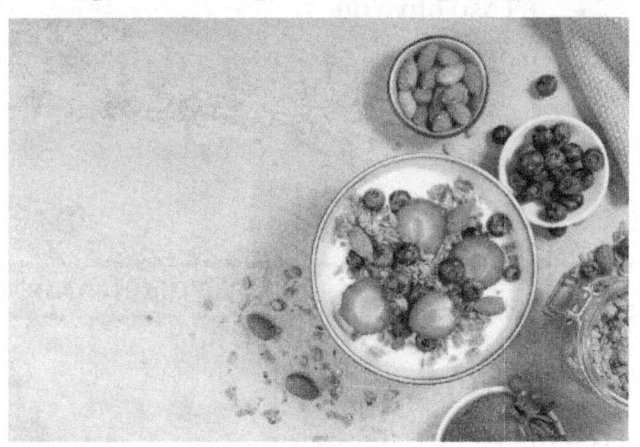

CHIA SEED PUDDING WITH ALMOND MILK

PREPARATION TIME: 5 min.
COOKING TIME: 0 min. (Chill overnight)
MODE OF COOKING: Refrigeration
INGREDIENTS:
- 1/4 cup chia seeds
- 1 cup unsweetened almond milk
- 1 Tbsp maple syrup
- 1/2 tsp vanilla extract
- Fresh berries for topping

DIRECTIONS:
1. In a bowl, whisk together chia seeds, almond milk, maple syrup, and vanilla extract.
2. Let it sit for 5 minutes, then stir again to prevent clumping.
3. Cover and refrigerate overnight.
4. Serve with fresh berries on top.

TIPS:
- Add a spoonful of nut butter for extra protein.
- Use coconut milk for a creamier texture.

NUTRITIONAL VALUES: Calories: 180, Fat: 10g, Carbs: 20g, Protein: 5g, Sugar: 8g

VEGETABLE AND EGG BREAKFAST MUFFINS

PREPARATION TIME: 10 min.
COOKING TIME: 25 min.
MODE OF COOKING: Baking
INGREDIENTS:
- 6 large eggs
- 1/2 cup bell peppers, diced
- 1/2 cup spinach, chopped
- 1/4 cup onion, diced
- 1/4 cup cherry tomatoes, halved
- 1/4 cup feta cheese, crumbled
- Salt and pepper to taste

DIRECTIONS:
1. Preheat oven to 350°F (175°C). Grease a muffin tin.
2. In a large bowl, whisk eggs and season with salt and pepper.
3. Stir in bell peppers, spinach, onion, and cherry tomatoes.
4. Pour the mixture evenly into the muffin tin cups.
5. Sprinkle feta cheese on top.
6. Bake for 20-25 minutes, until the muffins are set and slightly golden.

TIPS:
- Store leftovers in the refrigerator for a quick breakfast during the week.
- Add cooked bacon or sausage for extra protein.

NUTRITIONAL VALUES: Calories: 100, Fat: 7g, Carbs: 3g, Protein: 6g, Sugar: 1g

QUINOA BREAKFAST BOWL

PREPARATION TIME: 5 min.
COOKING TIME: 15 min.
MODE OF COOKING: Boiling
INGREDIENTS:
- 1/2 cup quinoa, rinsed
- 1 cup water
- 1/2 cup almond milk
- 1 banana, sliced
- 1/4 cup blueberries
- 1 Tbsp chia seeds
- 1 Tbsp almond butter
- 1 Tbsp honey

DIRECTIONS:
1. In a saucepan, bring quinoa and water to a boil. Reduce heat, cover, and simmer for 15 minutes, until water is absorbed.
2. Stir in almond milk and cook for an additional 2 minutes.
3. Divide quinoa into two bowls.

4. Top with banana slices, blueberries, chia seeds, and a drizzle of almond butter and honey.

TIPS:
- Prepare quinoa ahead of time and reheat for a quick breakfast.
- Substitute almond butter with peanut butter if preferred.

NUTRITIONAL VALUES: Calories: 350, Fat: 12g, Carbs: 52g, Protein: 10g, Sugar: 18g

SWEET POTATO AND AVOCADO TOAST

PREPARATION TIME: 5 min.
COOKING TIME: 10 min.
MODE OF COOKING: Toasting
INGREDIENTS:
- 1 large sweet potato, sliced lengthwise into 1/4 inch slices
- 1 ripe avocado, mashed
- 1/2 lemon, juiced
- Salt and pepper to taste
- Red pepper flakes (optional)

DIRECTIONS:
1. Toast sweet potato slices in a toaster or oven until tender and slightly crisp.
2. In a bowl, mash avocado with lemon juice, salt, and pepper.
3. Spread mashed avocado on sweet potato slices.
4. Sprinkle with red pepper flakes if desired.
5. Serve immediately.

TIPS:
- Add a poached egg on top for extra protein.
- Sprinkle with seeds like sesame or pumpkin for added texture.

NUTRITIONAL VALUES: Calories: 250, Fat: 15g, Carbs: 27g, Protein: 3g, Sugar: 5g

COCONUT YOGURT WITH PINEAPPLE AND ALMONDS

PREPARATION TIME: 5 min.
COOKING TIME: 0 min.
MODE OF COOKING: Assembling
INGREDIENTS:
- 2 cups coconut yogurt
- 1 cup fresh pineapple, diced
- 1/4 cup sliced almonds
- 1 Tbsp unsweetened shredded coconut
- 1 tsp chia seeds
- 1 Tbsp honey (optional)

DIRECTIONS:
1. In two bowls, divide the coconut yogurt.
2. Top with diced pineapple, sliced almonds, shredded coconut, and chia seeds.
3. Drizzle with honey if desired.
4. Serve immediately.

TIPS:
- Use Greek yogurt instead of coconut

yogurt for higher protein content.
- Add a handful of granola for extra crunch.

NUTRITIONAL VALUES: Calories: 220, Fat: 12g, Carbs: 22g, Protein: 5g, Sugar: 15g

ALMOND BUTTER AND BANANA SMOOTHIE

PREPARATION TIME: 5 min.
COOKING TIME: 0 min.
MODE OF COOKING: Blending
INGREDIENTS:
- 2 bananas, frozen
- 1 cup unsweetened almond milk
- 2 Tbsp almond butter
- 1 Tbsp chia seeds
- 1/2 tsp vanilla extract

DIRECTIONS:
1. In a blender, combine bananas, almond milk, almond butter, chia seeds, and vanilla extract.
2. Blend until smooth and creamy.
3. Pour into glasses and serve immediately.

TIPS:
- Add a handful of spinach for extra nutrients.
- Use peanut butter instead of almond butter for a different flavor.

NUTRITIONAL VALUES: Calories: 280, Fat: 12g, Carbs: 42g, Protein: 5g, Sugar: 20g

SAVORY OATMEAL WITH SPINACH AND EGG

PREPARATION TIME: 5 min.
COOKING TIME: 10 min.
MODE OF COOKING: Boiling
INGREDIENTS:
- 1 cup rolled oats
- 2 cups water
- 1 cup fresh spinach, chopped
- 1/4 cup feta cheese, crumbled
- 2 large eggs
- 1 Tbsp olive oil
- Salt and pepper to taste

DIRECTIONS:
1. In a saucepan, bring water to a boil. Add oats and reduce heat to a simmer. Cook for 5 minutes, stirring occasionally.
2. In a separate pan, heat olive oil over medium heat. Add spinach and sauté until wilted.
3. Stir spinach and feta cheese into the cooked oats. Season with salt and pepper.
4. In the same pan, fry the eggs to your liking.
5. Divide the oatmeal into two bowls and top each with a fried egg.

TIPS:
- Add a dash of hot sauce for extra flavor.
- Sprinkle with toasted nuts for added crunch.

NUTRITIONAL VALUES: Calories: 320, Fat: 16g, Carbs: 30g, Protein: 15g, Sugar: 2g

CHAPTER 4: LUNCHES

GRILLED CHICKEN AND QUINOA SALAD

PREPARATION TIME: 15 min.
COOKING TIME: 20 min.
MODE OF COOKING: Grilling and Boiling
INGREDIENTS:

- 2 boneless, skinless chicken breasts
- 1 cup quinoa, rinsed
- 2 cups water
- 1 cup cherry tomatoes, halved
- 1 cucumber, diced
- 1/4 cup red onion, finely chopped
- 1/4 cup feta cheese, crumbled
- 2 Tbsp olive oil
- Juice of 1 lemon
- 1 tsp dried oregano
- Salt and pepper to taste

DIRECTIONS:

1. Preheat grill to medium-high heat.
2. Season chicken breasts with salt, pepper, and dried oregano.
3. Grill chicken for 6-7 minutes on each side, or until fully cooked. Let it rest for 5 minutes before slicing.
4. In a saucepan, bring quinoa and water to a boil. Reduce heat, cover, and simmer for 15 minutes, or until water is absorbed.
5. In a large bowl, combine cooked quinoa, cherry tomatoes, cucumber, red onion, and feta cheese.
6. Drizzle with olive oil and lemon juice, then toss to combine.
7. Top with grilled chicken slices and serve.

TIPS:

- Add fresh herbs like parsley or mint for extra flavor.
- Serve with a side of mixed greens for added nutrients.

NUTRITIONAL VALUES: Calories: 350, Fat: 12g, Carbs: 32g, Protein: 28g, Sugar: 3g

TURKEY AND AVOCADO LETTUCE WRAPS

PREPARATION TIME: 10 min.
COOKING TIME: 0 min.
MODE OF COOKING: Assembling
INGREDIENTS:

- 8 large lettuce leaves
- 1/2 lb deli turkey breast, sliced
- 1 ripe avocado, sliced
- 1/4 cup red bell pepper, julienned
- 1/4 cup cucumber, julienned
- 1/4 cup shredded carrots
- 2 Tbsp hummus
- Salt and pepper to taste

DIRECTIONS:

1. Lay lettuce leaves flat on a clean surface.
2. Spread 1 tsp of hummus in the center of each leaf.
3. Layer turkey slices, avocado, bell

pepper, cucumber, and carrots on top of the hummus.
4. Season with salt and pepper.
5. Roll the lettuce leaves tightly to form wraps and secure with a toothpick if necessary.
6. Serve immediately.

TIPS:
- Use a variety of colored bell peppers for a vibrant presentation.
- Add a sprinkle of sunflower seeds for added crunch.

NUTRITIONAL VALUES: Calories: 250, Fat: 15g, Carbs: 12g, Protein: 22g, Sugar: 3g

SPINACH AND FETA STUFFED PEPPERS

PREPARATION TIME: 15 min.
COOKING TIME: 30 min.
MODE OF COOKING: Baking
INGREDIENTS:
- 4 bell peppers, halved and seeded
- 1 cup cooked quinoa
- 1 cup fresh spinach, chopped
- 1/2 cup feta cheese, crumbled
- 1/4 cup red onion, finely chopped
- 2 cloves garlic, minced
- 1 Tbsp olive oil
- Salt and pepper to taste

DIRECTIONS:
1. Preheat oven to 375°F (190°C).
2. In a skillet, heat olive oil over medium heat. Add red onion and garlic, sauté until fragrant.
3. Stir in chopped spinach and cook until wilted.
4. In a bowl, combine cooked quinoa, sautéed spinach mixture, and feta cheese. Season with salt and pepper.
5. Stuff each bell pepper half with the quinoa mixture.
6. Place stuffed peppers in a baking dish and bake for 25-30 minutes, until peppers are tender.

TIPS:
- Top with a sprinkle of shredded mozzarella before baking for extra cheesiness.
- Serve with a side of mixed greens or a simple cucumber salad.

NUTRITIONAL VALUES: Calories: 220, Fat: 10g, Carbs: 25g, Protein: 8g, Sugar: 5g

GRILLED SHRIMP TACOS WITH AVOCADO SALSA

PREPARATION TIME: 15 min.
COOKING TIME: 10 min.
MODE OF COOKING: Grilling
INGREDIENTS:
- 1 lb shrimp, peeled and deveined
- 1 Tbsp olive oil
- 1 tsp chili powder
- 1 tsp cumin
- 1/2 tsp garlic powder
- 1/4 tsp salt

- 8 small corn tortillas
- 1 avocado, diced
- 1/2 cup cherry tomatoes, quartered
- 1/4 cup red onion, finely chopped
- Juice of 1 lime
- 2 Tbsp cilantro, chopped

DIRECTIONS:
1. Preheat grill to medium-high heat.
2. In a bowl, toss shrimp with olive oil, chili powder, cumin, garlic powder, and salt.
3. Grill shrimp for 2-3 minutes on each side, until pink and opaque.
4. In a separate bowl, combine avocado, cherry tomatoes, red onion, lime juice, and cilantro to make the salsa.
5. Warm corn tortillas on the grill for about 30 seconds per side.
6. Assemble tacos by placing grilled shrimp on each tortilla and topping with avocado salsa.
7. Serve immediately.

TIPS:
- Add a dollop of Greek yogurt for a creamy texture.
- Serve with a side of black beans or rice.

NUTRITIONAL VALUES: Calories: 300, Fat: 15g, Carbs: 24g, Protein: 20g, Sugar: 2g

CHICKEN AND VEGETABLE STIR-FRY

PREPARATION TIME: 10 min.
COOKING TIME: 15 min.
MODE OF COOKING: Stir-Frying
INGREDIENTS:
- 2 boneless, skinless chicken breasts, sliced
- 1 red bell pepper, julienned
- 1 yellow bell pepper, julienned
- 1 cup broccoli florets
- 1 carrot, julienned
- 2 cloves garlic, minced
- 1 Tbsp ginger, minced
- 2 Tbsp soy sauce
- 1 Tbsp olive oil
- 1/4 cup green onions, sliced
- Salt and pepper to taste

DIRECTIONS:
1. Heat olive oil in a large skillet or wok over medium-high heat.
2. Add garlic and ginger, sauté until fragrant.
3. Add chicken slices and cook until browned and cooked through.
4. Add bell peppers, broccoli, and carrot to the skillet. Stir-fry until vegetables are tender-crisp.
5. Stir in soy sauce and cook for another 2 minutes.
6. Sprinkle with green onions before serving.

TIPS:
- Serve over brown rice or quinoa for a complete meal.

- Add a splash of sesame oil for extra flavor.

NUTRITIONAL VALUES: Calories: 280, Fat: 10g, Carbs: 15g, Protein: 30g, Sugar: 5g

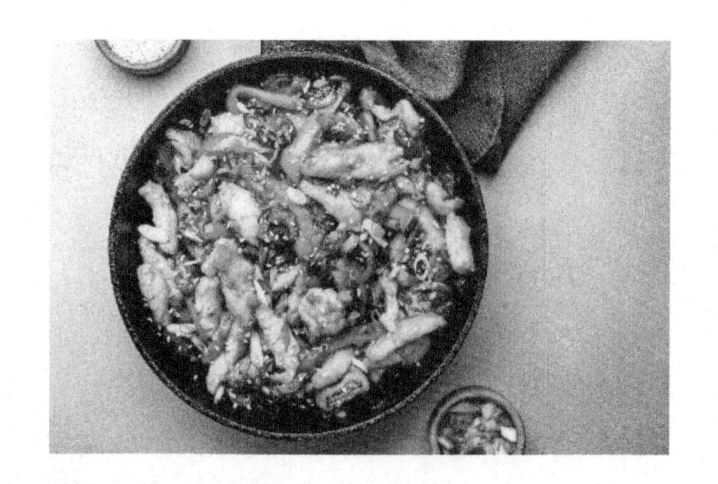

TUNA AND WHITE BEAN SALAD

PREPARATION TIME: 10 min.
COOKING TIME: 0 min.
MODE OF COOKING: Assembling
INGREDIENTS:

- 2 cans tuna in water, drained
- 1 can white beans, rinsed and drained
- 1/2 cup cherry tomatoes, halved
- 1/4 cup red onion, finely chopped
- 1/4 cup fresh parsley, chopped
- 2 Tbsp capers
- 3 Tbsp olive oil
- Juice of 1 lemon
- Salt and pepper to taste

DIRECTIONS:

1. In a large bowl, combine tuna, white beans, cherry tomatoes, red onion, parsley, and capers.
2. Drizzle with olive oil and lemon juice.
3. Season with salt and pepper to taste.
4. Toss well to combine and serve immediately.

TIPS:

- Add some baby arugula for a peppery flavor.
- Serve with whole grain crackers or bread.

NUTRITIONAL VALUES: Calories: 220, Fat: 12g, Carbs: 15g, Protein: 18g, Sugar: 2g

LENTIL AND KALE SOUP

PREPARATION TIME: 10 min.
COOKING TIME: 30 min.
MODE OF COOKING: Boiling
INGREDIENTS:

- 1 cup lentils, rinsed
- 6 cups vegetable broth
- 1 onion, diced
- 2 carrots, diced
- 2 celery stalks, diced
- 2 cloves garlic, minced
- 2 cups kale, chopped
- 1 can diced tomatoes
- 1 tsp dried thyme
- 1 tsp dried oregano

- 1 Tbsp olive oil
- Salt and pepper to taste

DIRECTIONS:
1. In a large pot, heat olive oil over medium heat. Add onion, carrots, and celery, sauté until tender.
2. Add garlic and cook for another minute.
3. Stir in lentils, vegetable broth, diced tomatoes, thyme, and oregano. Bring to a boil.
4. Reduce heat, cover, and simmer for 20 minutes, until lentils are tender.
5. Add chopped kale and cook for an additional 5 minutes.
6. Season with salt and pepper to taste.
7. Serve hot.

TIPS:
- Add a squeeze of lemon juice before serving for a fresh flavor.
- Serve with crusty whole grain bread.

NUTRITIONAL VALUES: Calories: 250, Fat: 5g, Carbs: 40g, Protein: 12g, Sugar: 6g

BALSAMIC CHICKEN AND VEGGIE SKEWERS

PREPARATION TIME: 20 min.
COOKING TIME: 15 min.
MODE OF COOKING: Grilling
INGREDIENTS:
- 2 boneless, skinless chicken breasts, cut into cubes
- 1 red bell pepper, cut into chunks
- 1 yellow bell pepper, cut into chunks
- 1 zucchini, sliced
- 1 red onion, cut into chunks
- 1/4 cup balsamic vinegar
- 2 Tbsp olive oil
- 1 tsp dried rosemary
- Salt and pepper to taste
- Skewers

DIRECTIONS:
1. Preheat grill to medium-high heat.
2. In a bowl, whisk together balsamic vinegar, olive oil, dried rosemary, salt, and pepper.
3. Thread chicken, bell peppers, zucchini, and red onion onto skewers.
4. Brush the balsamic mixture over the skewers.
5. Grill skewers for 12-15 minutes, turning occasionally, until chicken is fully cooked and vegetables are tender.
6. Serve immediately.

TIPS:
- Soak wooden skewers in water for 30 minutes before grilling to prevent burning.
- Serve with a side of quinoa or couscous.

NUTRITIONAL VALUES: Calories: 290, Fat: 12g, Carbs: 15g, Protein: 28g, Sugar: 7g

Quinoa and Black Bean Stuffed Sweet Potatoes

PREPARATION TIME: 10 min.
COOKING TIME: 45 min.
MODE OF COOKING: Baking
INGREDIENTS:

- 4 medium sweet potatoes
- 1 cup cooked quinoa
- 1 can black beans, rinsed and drained
- 1/2 cup corn kernels
- 1/4 cup red onion, diced
- 1/4 cup fresh cilantro, chopped
- 1 avocado, diced
- Juice of 1 lime
- 1 tsp cumin
- 1 tsp chili powder
- 2 Tbsp olive oil
- Salt and pepper to taste

DIRECTIONS:

1. Preheat oven to 400°F (200°C). Prick sweet potatoes with a fork and bake for 45 minutes, or until tender.
2. In a large bowl, combine cooked quinoa, black beans, corn, red onion, cilantro, cumin, chili powder, olive oil, and lime juice. Season with salt and pepper.
3. Once sweet potatoes are done, slice them open and fluff the insides with a fork.
4. Spoon the quinoa and black bean mixture into each sweet potato.
5. Top with diced avocado and serve immediately.

TIPS:

- Add a dollop of Greek yogurt for extra creaminess.
- Garnish with a sprinkle of feta cheese if desired.

NUTRITIONAL VALUES: Calories: 350, Fat: 14g, Carbs: 52g, Protein: 9g, Sugar: 9g

CHAPTER 5: DINNERS

LEMON HERB GRILLED SALMON

PREPARATION TIME: 10 min
COOKING TIME: 15 min
MODE OF COOKING: Grilling
INGREDIENTS:

- 4 salmon fillets
- 2 Tbsp olive oil
- 1 lemon, zested and juiced
- 2 cloves garlic, minced
- 1 tsp dried oregano
- 1 tsp dried thyme
- Salt and pepper to taste

DIRECTIONS:

1. Preheat grill to medium-high heat.
2. In a small bowl, whisk together olive oil, lemon zest, lemon juice, garlic, oregano, thyme, salt, and pepper.
3. Brush salmon fillets with the lemon herb mixture.
4. Grill salmon for 6-8 minutes on each side, or until fully cooked and flaky.
5. Serve immediately with a side of steamed vegetables or a fresh salad.

TIPS:

- Serve with a wedge of lemon for extra brightness.
- Add a sprinkle of fresh dill for added flavor.

NUTRITIONAL VALUES: Calories: 350, Fat: 18g, Carbs: 2g, Protein: 38g, Sugar: 0g

BAKED CHICKEN WITH ASPARAGUS AND TOMATOES

PREPARATION TIME: 10 min
COOKING TIME: 25 min
MODE OF COOKING: Baking
INGREDIENTS:

- 4 boneless, skinless chicken breasts
- 1 bunch asparagus, trimmed
- 1 pint cherry tomatoes
- 2 Tbsp olive oil
- 1 tsp garlic powder
- 1 tsp dried basil
- Salt and pepper to taste
- 1 lemon, sliced

DIRECTIONS:

1. Preheat oven to 400°F (200°C).
2. Place chicken breasts in a baking dish. Arrange asparagus and cherry tomatoes around the chicken.
3. Drizzle with olive oil and season with garlic powder, dried basil, salt, and pepper.
4. Top with lemon slices.
5. Bake for 25 minutes, or until chicken is fully cooked and vegetables are tender.
6. Serve immediately.

TIPS:

- Add a side of quinoa or brown rice for a complete meal.

- Garnish with fresh basil before serving.

NUTRITIONAL VALUES: Calories: 300, Fat: 12g, Carbs: 10g, Protein: 40g, Sugar: 4g

---

BEEF AND BROCCOLI STIR-FRY

PREPARATION TIME: 10 min
COOKING TIME: 15 min
MODE OF COOKING: Stir-Frying
INGREDIENTS:
- 1 lb flank steak, thinly sliced
- 1 head broccoli, cut into florets
- 2 cloves garlic, minced
- 1 Tbsp ginger, minced
- 3 Tbsp soy sauce
- 2 Tbsp oyster sauce
- 1 Tbsp olive oil
- 1 tsp sesame oil
- 1/4 cup green onions, sliced
- Salt and pepper to taste

DIRECTIONS:
1. Heat olive oil in a large skillet or wok over medium-high heat.
2. Add garlic and ginger, sauté until fragrant.
3. Add steak slices and cook until browned.
4. Add broccoli florets and stir-fry until tender-crisp.
5. Stir in soy sauce, oyster sauce, and sesame oil. Cook for another 2 minutes.
6. Sprinkle with green onions before serving.

TIPS:
- Serve over cauliflower rice for a low-carb option.
- Add a pinch of red pepper flakes for a spicy kick.

NUTRITIONAL VALUES: Calories: 320, Fat: 15g, Carbs: 12g, Protein: 36g, Sugar: 3g

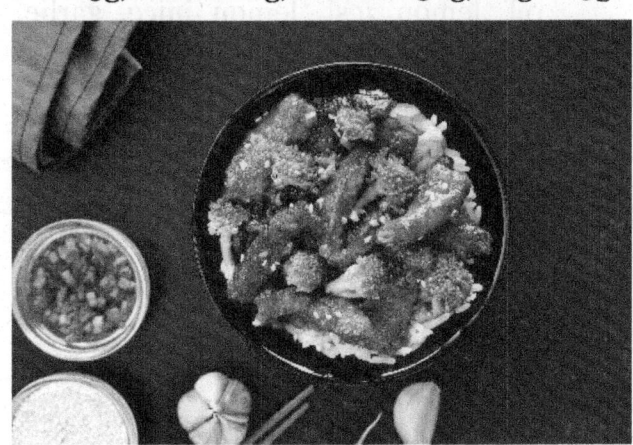

SHRIMP AND AVOCADO SALAD

PREPARATION TIME: 10 min
COOKING TIME: 5 min
MODE OF COOKING: Assembling
INGREDIENTS:
- 1 lb shrimp, peeled and deveined
- 1 avocado, diced
- 1 cup cherry tomatoes, halved
- 1/4 cup red onion, finely chopped
- 2 Tbsp fresh cilantro, chopped
- 2 Tbsp olive oil
- Juice of 1 lime
- Salt and pepper to taste

DIRECTIONS:
1. In a skillet, heat 1 Tbsp olive oil over medium heat. Add shrimp and cook until pink and opaque.
2. In a large bowl, combine cooked shrimp, avocado, cherry tomatoes, red onion, and cilantro.
3. Drizzle with remaining olive oil and lime juice. Season with salt and pepper.
4. Toss gently to combine and serve immediately.

TIPS:
- Serve on a bed of mixed greens for added volume.
- Add a sprinkle of feta cheese for extra flavor.

NUTRITIONAL VALUES: Calories: 280, Fat: 18g, Carbs: 10g, Protein: 22g, Sugar: 2g

LEMON GARLIC CHICKEN THIGHS

PREPARATION TIME: 10 min
COOKING TIME: 35 min
MODE OF COOKING: Baking
INGREDIENTS:
- 6 chicken thighs, bone-in, skin-on
- 3 cloves garlic, minced
- 1 lemon, juiced and zested
- 2 Tbsp olive oil
- 1 tsp dried oregano
- 1 tsp dried thyme
- Salt and pepper to taste

DIRECTIONS:
1. Preheat oven to 375°F (190°C).
2. In a small bowl, whisk together garlic, lemon juice, lemon zest, olive oil, oregano, thyme, salt, and pepper.
3. Place chicken thighs in a baking dish and pour the lemon garlic mixture over them.
4. Bake for 35 minutes, or until chicken is fully cooked and skin is crispy.
5. Serve immediately with your favorite side dish.

TIPS:
- Serve with roasted vegetables or a side salad.
- Garnish with fresh parsley for added color.

NUTRITIONAL VALUES: Calories: 400, Fat: 28g, Carbs: 2g, Protein: 35g, Sugar: 0g

STUFFED BELL PEPPERS WITH TURKEY AND QUINOA

PREPARATION TIME: 15 min
COOKING TIME: 30 min
MODE OF COOKING: Baking

INGREDIENTS:
- 4 bell peppers, halved and seeded
- 1 lb ground turkey
- 1 cup cooked quinoa

- 1/2 cup onion, diced
- 1/2 cup tomato sauce
- 1/2 cup shredded mozzarella cheese
- 2 cloves garlic, minced
- 1 Tbsp olive oil
- 1 tsp dried basil
- Salt and pepper to taste

DIRECTIONS:
1. Preheat oven to 375°F (190°C).
2. In a skillet, heat olive oil over medium heat. Add onion and garlic, sauté until tender.
3. Add ground turkey and cook until browned. Stir in cooked quinoa, tomato sauce, dried basil, salt, and pepper.
4. Fill each bell pepper half with the turkey mixture and place in a baking dish.
5. Sprinkle shredded mozzarella cheese on top.
6. Bake for 25-30 minutes, until peppers are tender and cheese is melted.
7. Serve immediately.

TIPS:
- Use different colored bell peppers for a vibrant presentation.
- Serve with a side of mixed greens.

NUTRITIONAL VALUES: Calories: 350, Fat: 15g, Carbs: 25g, Protein: 30g, Sugar: 6g

BALSAMIC GLAZED PORK CHOPS

PREPARATION TIME: 10 min
COOKING TIME: 20 min
MODE OF COOKING: Grilling
INGREDIENTS:
- 4 pork chops
- 1/4 cup balsamic vinegar
- 2 Tbsp olive oil
- 1 Tbsp honey
- 2 cloves garlic, minced
- Salt and pepper to taste

DIRECTIONS:
1. Preheat grill to medium-high heat.
2. In a small bowl, whisk together balsamic vinegar, olive oil, honey, garlic, salt, and pepper.
3. Brush pork chops with the balsamic glaze.
4. Grill pork chops for 5-7 minutes on each side, or until fully cooked.
5. Serve immediately with your favorite sides.

TIPS:
- Serve with roasted sweet potatoes and steamed vegetables.
- Garnish with fresh rosemary for added aroma.

NUTRITIONAL VALUES: Calories: 320, Fat: 20g, Carbs: 8g, Protein: 28g, Sugar: 6g

CAULIFLOWER RICE STIR-FRY WITH TOFU

PREPARATION TIME: 10 min
COOKING TIME: 15 min
MODE OF COOKING: Stir-Frying
INGREDIENTS:
- 1 block firm tofu, cubed
- 1 head cauliflower, riced
- 1 red bell pepper, diced
- 1 cup snap peas
- 2 cloves garlic, minced
- 1 Tbsp ginger, minced
- 3 Tbsp soy sauce
- 1 Tbsp sesame oil
- 1/4 cup green onions, sliced
- Salt and pepper to taste

DIRECTIONS:
1. Heat sesame oil in a large skillet or wok over medium-high heat.
2. Add garlic and ginger, sauté until fragrant.
3. Add tofu cubes and cook until golden brown.
4. Stir in cauliflower rice, bell pepper, and snap peas. Cook until vegetables are tender-crisp.
5. Add soy sauce and cook for another 2 minutes.
6. Sprinkle with green onions before serving.

TIPS:
- Add a splash of rice vinegar for extra tang.
- Serve with a side of steamed broccoli.

NUTRITIONAL VALUES: Calories: 280, Fat: 15g, Carbs: 18g, Protein: 18g, Sugar: 4g

LEMON HERB BAKED COD

PREPARATION TIME: 10 min
COOKING TIME: 20 min
MODE OF COOKING: Baking
INGREDIENTS:
- 4 cod fillets
- 2 Tbsp olive oil
- 2 cloves garlic, minced
- 1 lemon, zested and juiced
- 1 tsp dried thyme
- 1 tsp dried parsley
- Salt and pepper to taste

DIRECTIONS:
1. Preheat oven to 375°F (190°C).
2. In a small bowl, whisk together olive oil, garlic, lemon zest, lemon juice, thyme, parsley, salt, and pepper.
3. Place cod fillets in a baking dish and brush with the lemon herb mixture.
4. Bake for 15-20 minutes, or until cod is opaque and flakes easily with a fork.
5. Serve immediately with a side of steamed vegetables or a fresh salad.

TIPS:
- Serve with a wedge of lemon for extra brightness.
- Add a sprinkle of fresh dill for added flavor.

NUTRITIONAL VALUES: Calories: 250, Fat: 10g, Carbs: 2g, Protein: 36g, Sugar: 0g

MEDITERRANEAN STUFFED EGGPLANT

PREPARATION TIME: 15 min
COOKING TIME: 40 min
MODE OF COOKING: Baking
INGREDIENTS:

- 2 large eggplants, halved and hollowed out
- 1 lb ground lamb
- 1 cup cooked quinoa
- 1/2 cup onion, diced
- 1/2 cup tomatoes, diced
- 1/4 cup feta cheese, crumbled
- 2 cloves garlic, minced
- 2 Tbsp olive oil
- 1 tsp dried oregano
- Salt and pepper to taste

DIRECTIONS:

1. Preheat oven to 375°F (190°C).
2. In a skillet, heat olive oil over medium heat. Add onion and garlic, sauté until tender.
3. Add ground lamb and cook until browned. Stir in cooked quinoa, diced tomatoes, dried oregano, salt, and pepper.
4. Stuff each eggplant half with the lamb mixture and place in a baking dish.
5. Sprinkle crumbled feta cheese on top.
6. Bake for 35-40 minutes, until eggplants are tender.
7. Serve immediately.

TIPS:

- Use ground beef or turkey as an alternative to lamb.
- Garnish with fresh parsley or mint before serving.

NUTRITIONAL VALUES: Calories: 380, Fat: 20g, Carbs: 25g, Protein: 25g, Sugar: 6g

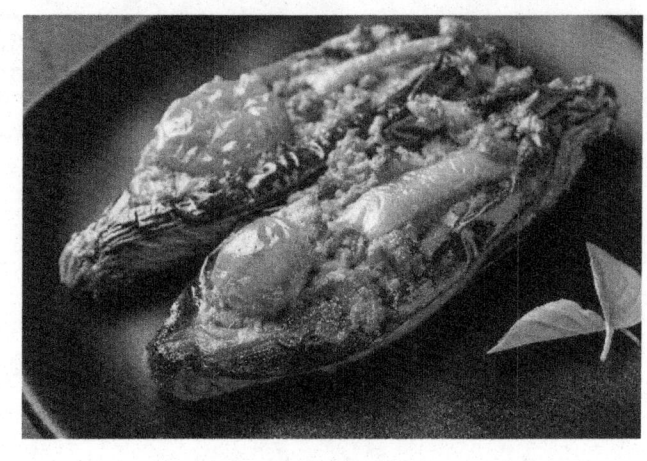

CHAPTER 6: SNACKS AND SIDES

SPICY ROASTED CHICKPEAS

PREPARATION TIME: 10 min
COOKING TIME: 40 min
MODE OF COOKING: Roasting
INGREDIENTS:

- 2 cans chickpeas, rinsed and drained
- 2 Tbsp olive oil
- 1 tsp smoked paprika
- 1/2 tsp cayenne pepper
- 1 tsp garlic powder
- 1/2 tsp salt

DIRECTIONS:

1. Preheat oven to 400°F (200°C).
2. Pat chickpeas dry with a paper towel.
3. In a large bowl, toss chickpeas with olive oil, smoked paprika, cayenne pepper, garlic powder, and salt.
4. Spread chickpeas evenly on a baking sheet.
5. Roast for 35-40 minutes, shaking the pan halfway through, until chickpeas are crispy.
6. Let cool before serving.

TIPS:

- Store in an airtight container for up to a week.
- Add a squeeze of lemon juice for extra flavor.

NUTRITIONAL VALUES: Calories: 150, Fat: 7g, Carbs: 18g, Protein: 5g, Sugar: 1g

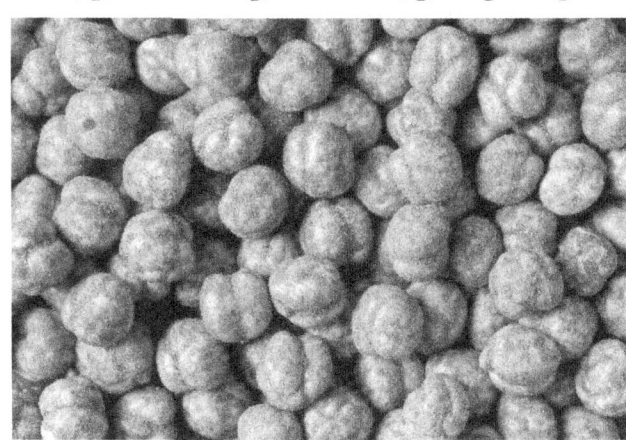

GREEK YOGURT AND CUCUMBER DIP

PREPARATION TIME: 10 min
COOKING TIME: 0 min
MODE OF COOKING: Assembling
INGREDIENTS:

- 1 cup Greek yogurt
- 1/2 cucumber, grated
- 1 clove garlic, minced
- 1 Tbsp fresh dill, chopped
- Juice of 1/2 lemon
- Salt and pepper to taste

DIRECTIONS:

1. In a medium bowl, combine Greek yogurt, grated cucumber, garlic, dill, lemon juice, salt, and pepper.
2. Mix well until all ingredients are thoroughly combined.
3. Serve immediately or refrigerate for up to 2 days.

TIPS:

- Serve with vegetable sticks or whole-grain crackers.

- Add a drizzle of olive oil on top for extra richness.

NUTRITIONAL VALUES: Calories: 80, Fat: 2g, Carbs: 5g, Protein: 10g, Sugar: 4g

BAKED ZUCCHINI FRIES

PREPARATION TIME: 10 min
COOKING TIME: 25 min
MODE OF COOKING: Baking
INGREDIENTS:
- 2 large zucchinis, cut into fries
- 1/2 cup almond flour
- 1/4 cup grated Parmesan cheese
- 1 tsp garlic powder
- 1 tsp Italian seasoning
- 1/2 tsp salt
- 1/2 tsp black pepper
- 1 egg, beaten

DIRECTIONS:
1. Preheat oven to 425°F (220°C). Line a baking sheet with parchment paper.
2. In a shallow dish, mix almond flour, Parmesan cheese, garlic powder, Italian seasoning, salt, and pepper.
3. Dip each zucchini fry in the beaten egg, then coat with the almond flour mixture.
4. Place coated zucchini fries on the prepared baking sheet.
5. Bake for 20-25 minutes, until golden and crispy.
6. Serve immediately with your favorite dipping sauce.

TIPS:
- Serve with marinara sauce for a tasty pairing.
- Sprinkle with extra Parmesan before serving.

NUTRITIONAL VALUES: Calories: 120, Fat: 8g, Carbs: 6g, Protein: 7g, Sugar: 2g

AVOCADO DEVILED EGGS

PREPARATION TIME: 10 min
COOKING TIME: 10 min
MODE OF COOKING: Boiling and Assembling
INGREDIENTS:
- 6 large eggs
- 1 ripe avocado
- 1 Tbsp Greek yogurt
- 1 tsp lime juice
- 1/2 tsp garlic powder
- Salt and pepper to taste
- Paprika for garnish

DIRECTIONS:
1. Place eggs in a saucepan and cover with water. Bring to a boil, then remove from heat and let sit for 10 minutes.
2. Drain and cool eggs under cold running water. Peel the eggs and slice in half lengthwise.

3. Scoop out the yolks into a bowl and mash with avocado, Greek yogurt, lime juice, garlic powder, salt, and pepper.
4. Spoon or pipe the avocado mixture back into the egg whites.
5. Garnish with a sprinkle of paprika before serving.

TIPS:
- Add a dash of hot sauce for a spicy kick.
- Store leftovers in the refrigerator for up to 2 days.

NUTRITIONAL VALUES: Calories: 90, Fat: 7g, Carbs: 3g, Protein: 6g, Sugar: 1g

GARLIC AND HERB CAULIFLOWER MASH

PREPARATION TIME: 10 min
COOKING TIME: 15 min
MODE OF COOKING: Boiling
INGREDIENTS:
- 1 large head of cauliflower, cut into florets
- 2 cloves garlic, minced
- 2 Tbsp olive oil
- 1/4 cup unsweetened almond milk
- 1 tsp dried thyme
- Salt and pepper to taste

DIRECTIONS:
1. Bring a large pot of salted water to a boil. Add cauliflower florets and cook until tender, about 10 minutes.
2. Drain cauliflower and transfer to a food processor.
3. Add garlic, olive oil, almond milk, thyme, salt, and pepper. Blend until smooth and creamy.
4. Serve immediately.

TIPS:
- Top with fresh chives for added flavor.
- Serve as a side dish with grilled meats.

NUTRITIONAL VALUES: Calories: 100, Fat: 8g, Carbs: 7g, Protein: 2g, Sugar: 2g

SPICY EDAMAME

PREPARATION TIME: 5 min
COOKING TIME: 5 min
MODE OF COOKING: Boiling and Sautéing
INGREDIENTS:
- 2 cups frozen edamame in pods
- 1 Tbsp soy sauce
- 1 tsp sesame oil
- 1/2 tsp red pepper flakes
- 1 clove garlic, minced

DIRECTIONS:
1. Bring a large pot of salted water to a boil. Add edamame and cook for 5 minutes. Drain.
2. In a skillet, heat sesame oil over medium heat. Add garlic and red pepper flakes, sauté until fragrant.
3. Add cooked edamame and soy sauce, toss to coat.
4. Serve immediately.

TIPS:
- Sprinkle with sesame seeds for added texture.
- Serve as an appetizer or side dish.

NUTRITIONAL VALUES: Calories: 120, Fat: 5g, Carbs: 9g, Protein: 9g, Sugar: 1g

Sweet Potato Chips

PREPARATION TIME: 10 min
COOKING TIME: 20 min
MODE OF COOKING: Baking
INGREDIENTS:
- 2 large sweet potatoes, thinly sliced
- 2 Tbsp olive oil
- 1 tsp paprika
- 1/2 tsp garlic powder
- Salt and pepper to taste

DIRECTIONS:
1. Preheat oven to 400°F (200°C). Line a baking sheet with parchment paper.
2. In a large bowl, toss sweet potato slices with olive oil, paprika, garlic powder, salt, and pepper.
3. Spread slices evenly on the prepared baking sheet.
4. Bake for 15-20 minutes, until crispy, flipping halfway through.
5. Serve immediately.

TIPS:
- Serve with a Greek yogurt dip.
- Sprinkle with fresh rosemary for added flavor.

NUTRITIONAL VALUES: Calories: 150, Fat: 7g, Carbs: 20g, Protein: 2g, Sugar: 4g

Roasted Brussels Sprouts with Balsamic Glaze

PREPARATION TIME: 10 min
COOKING TIME: 25 min
MODE OF COOKING: Roasting
INGREDIENTS:
- 1 lb Brussels sprouts, halved
- 2 Tbsp olive oil
- 1 Tbsp balsamic vinegar
- 1 Tbsp honey
- Salt and pepper to taste

DIRECTIONS:
1. Preheat oven to 400°F (200°C).
2. In a large bowl, toss Brussels sprouts with olive oil, salt, and pepper.
3. Spread on a baking sheet and roast for 20 minutes, until tender and crispy.
4. In a small bowl, mix balsamic vinegar and honey. Drizzle over roasted Brussels sprouts.
5. Serve immediately.

TIPS:
- Add a sprinkle of Parmesan cheese before serving.
- Serve as a side dish with grilled chicken or fish.

NUTRITIONAL VALUES: Calories: 120, Fat: 7g, Carbs: 12g, Protein: 3g, Sugar: 6g

Garlic Parmesan Kale Chips

PREPARATION TIME: 10 min
COOKING TIME: 15 min
MODE OF COOKING: Baking
INGREDIENTS:
- 1 bunch kale, washed and torn into pieces
- 2 Tbsp olive oil
- 1/4 cup grated Parmesan cheese
- 1 tsp garlic powder
- Salt to taste

DIRECTIONS:
1. Preheat oven to 350°F (175°C). Line a baking sheet with parchment paper.
2. In a large bowl, toss kale with olive oil, Parmesan cheese, garlic powder, and salt.
3. Spread kale evenly on the prepared baking sheet.
4. Bake for 12-15 minutes, until crispy.
5. Serve immediately.

TIPS:
- Add a pinch of red pepper flakes for a spicy kick.
- Store in an airtight container for up to 3 days.

NUTRITIONAL VALUES: Calories: 100, Fat: 7g, Carbs: 7g, Protein: 4g, Sugar: 0g

Guacamole and Veggie Sticks

PREPARATION TIME: 10 min
COOKING TIME: 0 min
MODE OF COOKING: Assembling
INGREDIENTS:
- 2 ripe avocados, mashed
- 1/4 cup red onion, finely chopped
- 1 clove garlic, minced
- 1 tomato, diced
- Juice of 1 lime
- Salt and pepper to taste
- Assorted veggie sticks (carrots, celery, bell peppers)

DIRECTIONS:
1. In a medium bowl, combine mashed avocados, red onion, garlic, tomato, lime juice, salt, and pepper.
2. Mix well until all ingredients are thoroughly combined.
3. Serve immediately with assorted veggie sticks.

TIPS:
- Add chopped cilantro for extra flavor.
- Serve as a snack or appetizer.

NUTRITIONAL VALUES: Calories: 150, Fat: 12g, Carbs: 10g, Protein: 2g, Sugar: 2g

CHAPTER 7: DESSERTS

CHOCOLATE AVOCADO MOUSSE

PREPARATION TIME: 10 min
COOKING TIME: 0 min
MODE OF COOKING: Blending
INGREDIENTS:
- 2 ripe avocados
- 1/4 cup cocoa powder
- 1/4 cup honey or maple syrup
- 1/4 cup almond milk
- 1 tsp vanilla extract
- Pinch of salt

DIRECTIONS:
1. Scoop the flesh of the avocados into a blender.
2. Add cocoa powder, honey or maple syrup, almond milk, vanilla extract, and salt.
3. Blend until smooth and creamy.
4. Spoon into serving bowls and chill in the refrigerator for at least 1 hour before serving.

TIPS:
- Top with fresh berries or chopped nuts for extra texture.
- Use coconut milk for a richer flavor.

NUTRITIONAL VALUES: Calories: 220, Fat: 14g, Carbs: 24g, Protein: 3g, Sugar: 16g

BERRY CHIA PUDDING

PREPARATION TIME: 5 min
COOKING TIME: 0 min (Chill overnight)
MODE OF COOKING: Refrigeration
INGREDIENTS:
- 1/4 cup chia seeds
- 1 cup unsweetened almond milk
- 1 Tbsp honey or maple syrup
- 1/2 tsp vanilla extract
- 1/2 cup mixed berries

DIRECTIONS:
1. In a bowl, mix chia seeds, almond milk, honey or maple syrup, and vanilla extract.
2. Stir well to combine.
3. Cover and refrigerate overnight or for at least 4 hours until the mixture thickens.
4. Serve with mixed berries on top.

TIPS:
- Add a dollop of Greek yogurt for extra protein.
- Use any type of milk you prefer.

NUTRITIONAL VALUES: Calories: 180, Fat: 9g, Carbs: 21g, Protein: 4g, Sugar: 12g

ALMOND BUTTER BANANA BITES

PREPARATION TIME: 5 min
COOKING TIME: 0 min
MODE OF COOKING: Assembling
INGREDIENTS:
- 2 bananas, sliced into rounds
- 1/4 cup almond butter
- 2 Tbsp dark chocolate chips, melted

DIRECTIONS:
1. Spread a small amount of almond butter on half of the banana slices.
2. Top with the remaining banana slices to make sandwiches.
3. Drizzle with melted dark chocolate.
4. Chill in the refrigerator for 10 minutes before serving.

TIPS:
- Sprinkle with sea salt for a sweet and salty flavor.
- Use peanut butter instead of almond butter if preferred.

NUTRITIONAL VALUES: Calories: 150, Fat: 9g, Carbs: 18g, Protein: 3g, Sugar: 9g

COCONUT MACAROONS

PREPARATION TIME: 10 min
COOKING TIME: 20 min
MODE OF COOKING: Baking
INGREDIENTS:
- 2 cups shredded unsweetened coconut
- 1/4 cup honey or maple syrup
- 2 egg whites
- 1 tsp vanilla extract
- Pinch of salt

DIRECTIONS:
1. Preheat oven to 325°F (165°C). Line a baking sheet with parchment paper.
2. In a large bowl, mix shredded coconut, honey or maple syrup, egg whites, vanilla extract, and salt until well combined.
3. Scoop tablespoons of the mixture onto the prepared baking sheet.
4. Bake for 18-20 minutes, until golden brown.
5. Let cool before serving.

TIPS:
- Drizzle with melted dark chocolate for an extra treat.
- Store in an airtight container for up to a week.

NUTRITIONAL VALUES: Calories: 120, Fat: 8g, Carbs: 10g, Protein: 2g, Sugar: 7g

GREEK YOGURT AND BERRY POPSICLES

PREPARATION TIME: 10 min
COOKING TIME: 0 min (Freeze for 4 hours)
MODE OF COOKING: Freezing
INGREDIENTS:
- 1 cup Greek yogurt

- 1/2 cup mixed berries
- 2 Tbsp honey or maple syrup
- 1 tsp vanilla extract

DIRECTIONS:
1. In a blender, combine Greek yogurt, mixed berries, honey or maple syrup, and vanilla extract. Blend until smooth.
2. Pour the mixture into popsicle molds.
3. Freeze for at least 4 hours, until solid.
4. To remove, run the molds under warm water for a few seconds.

TIPS:
- Add chunks of fresh fruit to the molds before pouring the mixture for added texture.
- Use any type of fruit you prefer.

NUTRITIONAL VALUES: Calories: 80, Fat: 2g, Carbs: 11g, Protein: 4g, Sugar: 8g

DARK CHOCOLATE AND ALMOND CLUSTERS

PREPARATION TIME: 5 min
COOKING TIME: 5 min (Chill for 30 minutes)
MODE OF COOKING: Melting and Refrigeration
INGREDIENTS:
- 1 cup dark chocolate chips
- 1 cup whole almonds
- 1/2 tsp sea salt

DIRECTIONS:
1. Melt dark chocolate chips in a microwave or double boiler until smooth.
2. Stir in whole almonds until well coated.
3. Drop spoonfuls of the mixture onto a parchment-lined baking sheet.
4. Sprinkle with sea salt.
5. Chill in the refrigerator for at least 30 minutes until set.

TIPS:
- Add dried fruit like cranberries or raisins for extra sweetness.
- Store in an airtight container in the refrigerator.

NUTRITIONAL VALUES: Calories: 150, Fat: 10g, Carbs: 15g, Protein: 3g, Sugar: 10g

BAKED APPLE CHIPS

PREPARATION TIME: 10 min
COOKING TIME: 2 hours
MODE OF COOKING: Baking
INGREDIENTS:
- 2 apples, thinly sliced
- 1 tsp cinnamon
- 1 Tbsp coconut sugar (optional)

DIRECTIONS:
1. Preheat oven to 225°F (110°C). Line a baking sheet with parchment paper.
2. Arrange apple slices on the baking sheet in a single layer.

3. Sprinkle with cinnamon and coconut sugar, if using.
4. Bake for 2 hours, flipping halfway through, until crisp.
5. Let cool before serving.

TIPS:
- Store in an airtight container for up to a week.
- Use different types of apples for varied flavor.

NUTRITIONAL VALUES: Calories: 60, Fat: 0g, Carbs: 16g, Protein: 0g, Sugar: 12g

Lemon Blueberry Muffins

PREPARATION TIME: 15 min
COOKING TIME: 20 min
MODE OF COOKING: Baking
INGREDIENTS:
- 1 1/2 cups almond flour
- 1/2 cup coconut flour
- 1/4 cup honey or maple syrup
- 3 large eggs
- 1/3 cup coconut oil, melted
- 1/2 cup unsweetened almond milk
- 1 cup blueberries
- Zest of 1 lemon
- 1 tsp baking powder
- 1 tsp vanilla extract
- Pinch of salt

DIRECTIONS:
1. Preheat oven to 350°F (175°C). Line a muffin tin with paper liners.
2. In a large bowl, mix almond flour, coconut flour, baking powder, and salt.
3. In another bowl, whisk together eggs, honey or maple syrup, coconut oil, almond milk, lemon zest, and vanilla extract.
4. Combine wet and dry ingredients until just mixed. Fold in blueberries.
5. Divide the batter evenly among the muffin cups.
6. Bake for 18-20 minutes, until a toothpick inserted into the center comes out clean.
7. Let cool before serving.

TIPS:
- Add a lemon glaze made from lemon juice and powdered erythritol for extra sweetness.
- Store in an airtight container for up to 3 days.

NUTRITIONAL VALUES: Calories: 180, Fat: 12g, Carbs: 14g, Protein: 5g, Sugar: 8g

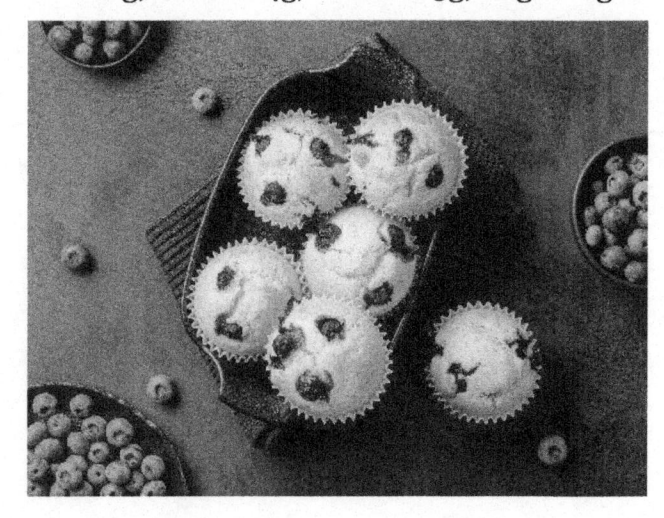

STRAWBERRY COCONUT ENERGY BALLS

PREPARATION TIME: 10 min
COOKING TIME: 0 min
MODE OF COOKING: No-Cook
INGREDIENTS:
- 1 cup dried strawberries
- 1 cup shredded unsweetened coconut
- 1/2 cup almond flour
- 2 Tbsp honey or maple syrup
- 1 tsp vanilla extract
- 1/4 cup coconut oil, melted

DIRECTIONS:
1. In a food processor, combine dried strawberries, shredded coconut, almond flour, honey or maple syrup, vanilla extract, and melted coconut oil.
2. Pulse until the mixture comes together.
3. Roll the mixture into small balls.
4. Chill in the refrigerator for 30 minutes before serving.

TIPS:
- Roll in extra shredded coconut for a prettier presentation.
- Store in an airtight container in the refrigerator.

NUTRITIONAL VALUES: Calories: 120, Fat: 8g, Carbs: 12g, Protein: 2g, Sugar: 8g

PUMPKIN SPICE LATTE SMOOTHIE

PREPARATION TIME: 5 min
COOKING TIME: 0 min
MODE OF COOKING: Blending
INGREDIENTS:
- 1 cup unsweetened almond milk
- 1/2 cup pumpkin puree
- 1 frozen banana
- 1/4 cup Greek yogurt
- 1 Tbsp honey or maple syrup
- 1 tsp pumpkin pie spice
- 1/2 tsp vanilla extract
- 1/4 cup brewed coffee, cooled

DIRECTIONS:
1. In a blender, combine almond milk, pumpkin puree, frozen banana, Greek yogurt, honey or maple syrup, pumpkin pie spice, vanilla extract, and brewed coffee.
2. Blend until smooth and creamy.
3. Pour into glasses and serve immediately.

TIPS:
- Top with a sprinkle of cinnamon for extra flavor.
- Use cold brew coffee for a stronger coffee flavor.

NUTRITIONAL VALUES: Calories: 150, Fat: 3g, Carbs: 27g, Protein: 5g, Sugar: 16g

CHAPTER 8: REFRESHING BEVERAGES

CUCUMBER MINT SPARKLER

PREPARATION TIME: 10 min
COOKING TIME: 0 min
MODE OF COOKING: Mixing
INGREDIENTS:

- 1 cucumber, thinly sliced
- 1/4 cup fresh mint leaves
- 1 quart sparkling water
- 1 lime, juiced
- 1 Tbsp honey or maple syrup (optional)
- Ice cubes

DIRECTIONS:

1. In a large pitcher, combine cucumber slices and mint leaves.
2. Add lime juice and honey or maple syrup if using.
3. Pour in sparkling water and stir gently.
4. Fill glasses with ice cubes and pour the cucumber mint sparkler over the ice.
5. Garnish with additional mint leaves and cucumber slices if desired.
6. Serve immediately.

TIPS:

- For a stronger mint flavor, muddle the mint leaves before adding.
- Use flavored sparkling water for a twist.

NUTRITIONAL VALUES: Calories: 10, Fat: 0g, Carbs: 2g, Protein: 0g, Sugar: 1g

TROPICAL GREEN SMOOTHIE

PREPARATION TIME: 5 min
COOKING TIME: 0 min
MODE OF COOKING: Blending
INGREDIENTS:

- 1 cup fresh spinach
- 1/2 cup frozen mango chunks
- 1/2 cup frozen pineapple chunks
- 1 banana
- 1 cup coconut water
- 1 Tbsp chia seeds

DIRECTIONS:

1. In a blender, combine spinach, mango, pineapple, banana, coconut water, and chia seeds.
2. Blend until smooth and creamy.
3. Pour into glasses and serve immediately.

TIPS:

- Add a scoop of protein powder for an extra protein boost.
- Garnish with a slice of pineapple or a sprinkle of chia seeds.

NUTRITIONAL VALUES: Calories: 150, Fat: 2g, Carbs: 34g, Protein: 3g, Sugar: 22g

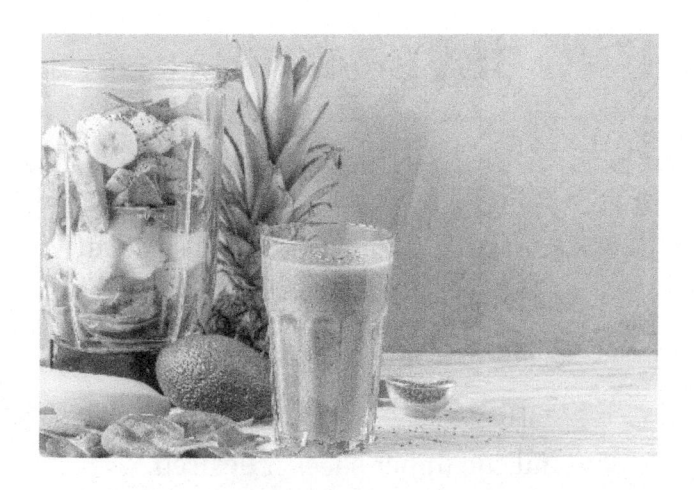

LEMON GINGER INFUSED WATER

PREPARATION TIME: 5 min
COOKING TIME: 0 min (Infuse for 1 hour)
MODE OF COOKING: Infusing
INGREDIENTS:

- 1 lemon, thinly sliced
- 1-inch piece of ginger, sliced
- 1 quart water
- Ice cubes

DIRECTIONS:

1. In a large pitcher, combine lemon slices and ginger slices.
2. Fill the pitcher with water.
3. Let it infuse in the refrigerator for at least 1 hour.
4. Fill glasses with ice cubes and pour the infused water over the ice.
5. Serve immediately.

TIPS:

- Add a few fresh mint leaves for extra flavor.
- Store in the refrigerator for up to 2 days.

NUTRITIONAL VALUES: Calories: 5, Fat: 0g, Carbs: 1g, Protein: 0g, Sugar: 0g

BERRY HIBISCUS ICED TEA

PREPARATION TIME: 5 min
COOKING TIME: 5 min
MODE OF COOKING: Steeping
INGREDIENTS:

- 4 hibiscus tea bags
- 1 cup mixed berries (strawberries, blueberries, raspberries)
- 4 cups boiling water
- 1 Tbsp honey or maple syrup (optional)
- Ice cubes

DIRECTIONS:

1. In a heatproof pitcher, add hibiscus tea bags and mixed berries.
2. Pour boiling water over the tea bags and berries.
3. Let steep for 5 minutes, then remove the tea bags.
4. Stir in honey or maple syrup if using.
5. Fill glasses with ice cubes and pour the

hibiscus tea over the ice.
6. Serve immediately.

TIPS:
- Garnish with extra berries and a sprig of mint.
- Use frozen berries to keep the drink extra cold.

NUTRITIONAL VALUES: Calories: 20, Fat: 0g, Carbs: 5g, Protein: 0g, Sugar: 4g

WATERMELON BASIL COOLER

PREPARATION TIME: 10 min
COOKING TIME: 0 min
MODE OF COOKING: Blending
INGREDIENTS:
- 4 cups watermelon, cubed
- 1/4 cup fresh basil leaves
- Juice of 1 lime
- 1 cup sparkling water
- Ice cubes

DIRECTIONS:
1. In a blender, combine watermelon, basil leaves, and lime juice. Blend until smooth.
2. Pour the mixture through a fine mesh strainer into a pitcher to remove the pulp.
3. Stir in sparkling water.
4. Fill glasses with ice cubes and pour the watermelon basil cooler over the ice.
5. Serve immediately.

TIPS:
- Add a splash of coconut water for extra hydration.
- Garnish with basil leaves and a watermelon wedge.

NUTRITIONAL VALUES: Calories: 30, Fat: 0g, Carbs: 8g, Protein: 0g, Sugar: 6g

PINEAPPLE MINT DETOX DRINK

PREPARATION TIME: 10 min
COOKING TIME: 0 min
MODE OF COOKING: Blending
INGREDIENTS:
- 1 cup fresh pineapple chunks
- 1/2 cucumber, sliced
- 1/4 cup fresh mint leaves
- Juice of 1 lemon
- 2 cups cold water
- Ice cubes

DIRECTIONS:
1. In a blender, combine pineapple, cucumber, mint leaves, lemon juice, and cold water. Blend until smooth.
2. Pour the mixture through a fine mesh strainer into a pitcher.
3. Fill glasses with ice cubes and pour the detox drink over the ice.
4. Serve immediately.

TIPS:
- Add a slice of ginger for an extra kick.
- Garnish with a cucumber slice and mint leaves.

NUTRITIONAL VALUES: Calories: 25, Fat: 0g, Carbs: 6g, Protein: 0g, Sugar: 4g

ICED MATCHA LATTE

PREPARATION TIME: 5 min
COOKING TIME: 0 min
MODE OF COOKING: Mixing
INGREDIENTS:
- 1 tsp matcha green tea powder
- 1 cup unsweetened almond milk
- 1 Tbsp honey or maple syrup (optional)
- Ice cubes

DIRECTIONS:
1. In a small bowl, whisk matcha green tea powder with a little bit of hot water to make a smooth paste.
2. In a glass, combine matcha paste, almond milk, and honey or maple syrup if using. Stir well.
3. Fill the glass with ice cubes.
4. Serve immediately.

TIPS:
- Use a matcha whisk for best results.
- Add a dash of vanilla extract for extra flavor.

NUTRITIONAL VALUES: Calories: 50, Fat: 2g, Carbs: 7g, Protein: 1g, Sugar: 5g

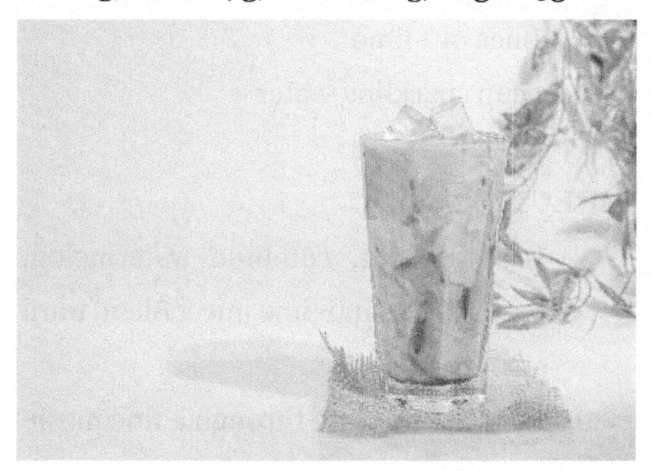

COCONUT LIME COOLER

PREPARATION TIME: 5 min
COOKING TIME: 0 min
MODE OF COOKING: Blending
INGREDIENTS:
- 1 cup coconut water
- 1/2 cup coconut milk
- Juice of 2 limes
- 1 Tbsp honey or maple syrup (optional)
- Ice cubes

DIRECTIONS:
1. In a blender, combine coconut water, coconut milk, lime juice, and honey or maple syrup if using. Blend until smooth.
2. Fill glasses with ice cubes and pour the coconut lime cooler over the ice.
3. Serve immediately.

TIPS:
- Garnish with a lime slice and a sprig of mint.
- Use sparkling water instead of coconut water for a fizzy drink.

NUTRITIONAL VALUES: Calories: 60, Fat: 3g, Carbs: 8g, Protein: 0g, Sugar: 7g

BERRY LEMONADE

PREPARATION TIME: 10 min
COOKING TIME: 0 min
MODE OF COOKING: Mixing
INGREDIENTS:
- 1 cup mixed berries (strawberries, blueberries, raspberries)
- Juice of 4 lemons
- 1/4 cup honey or maple syrup
- 4 cups cold water
- Ice cubes

DIRECTIONS:
1. In a blender, puree mixed berries until smooth.
2. In a pitcher, combine berry puree, lemon juice, honey or maple syrup, and cold water. Stir well.
3. Fill glasses with ice cubes and pour the berry lemonade over the ice.
4. Serve immediately.

TIPS:
- Garnish with fresh berries and a lemon slice.
- Add a few mint leaves for a refreshing twist.

NUTRITIONAL VALUES: Calories: 40, Fat: 0g, Carbs: 10g, Protein: 0g, Sugar: 8g

TURMERIC GINGER TEA

PREPARATION TIME: 5 min
COOKING TIME: 10 min
MODE OF COOKING: Boiling
INGREDIENTS:
- 1 tsp ground turmeric
- 1-inch piece of ginger, sliced
- 2 cups water
- Juice of 1 lemon
- 1 Tbsp honey or maple syrup

DIRECTIONS:
1. In a small saucepan, bring water, turmeric, and ginger to a boil.
2. Reduce heat and simmer for 10 minutes.
3. Strain the tea into a cup.
4. Stir in lemon juice and honey or maple syrup.
5. Serve hot or chilled over ice.

TIPS:
- Add a pinch of black pepper to enhance the absorption of turmeric.
- Store in the refrigerator for up to 2 days.

NUTRITIONAL VALUES: Calories: 30, Fat: 0g, Carbs: 8g, Protein: 0g, Sugar: 7g

CHAPTER 9: FISH AND SEAFOOD DELIGHTS

Garlic Butter Shrimp

PREPARATION TIME: 10 min
COOKING TIME: 10 min
MODE OF COOKING: Sautéing
INGREDIENTS:
- 1 lb shrimp, peeled and deveined
- 3 Tbsp butter
- 4 cloves garlic, minced
- Juice of 1 lemon
- 1 Tbsp fresh parsley, chopped
- Salt and pepper to taste

DIRECTIONS:
1. In a large skillet, melt butter over medium heat.
2. Add garlic and sauté until fragrant.
3. Add shrimp and cook until pink and opaque, about 2-3 minutes per side.
4. Stir in lemon juice and season with salt and pepper.
5. Sprinkle with fresh parsley and serve immediately.

TIPS:
- Serve over zucchini noodles or cauliflower rice for a low-carb option.
- Garnish with extra lemon wedges.

NUTRITIONAL VALUES: Calories: 200, Fat: 12g, Carbs: 2g, Protein: 20g, Sugar: 0g

Blackened Salmon

PREPARATION TIME: 5 min
COOKING TIME: 10 min
MODE OF COOKING: Pan-Searing
INGREDIENTS:
- 4 salmon fillets
- 2 Tbsp olive oil
- 2 tsp paprika
- 1 tsp cayenne pepper
- 1 tsp garlic powder
- 1 tsp onion powder
- 1 tsp dried thyme
- Salt and pepper to taste

DIRECTIONS:
1. In a small bowl, mix paprika, cayenne pepper, garlic powder, onion powder, thyme, salt, and pepper.
2. Rub the spice mixture evenly over both sides of the salmon fillets.
3. Heat olive oil in a large skillet over medium-high heat.
4. Add salmon and cook for 3-4 minutes per side, until blackened and fully cooked.
5. Serve immediately with a side of steamed vegetables or a fresh salad.

TIPS:
- Serve with a cooling yogurt sauce to balance the heat.
- Garnish with fresh cilantro.

NUTRITIONAL VALUES: Calories: 300, Fat: 20g, Carbs: 1g, Protein: 28g, Sugar: 0g

BAKED TILAPIA WITH CHERRY TOMATOES

PREPARATION TIME: 10 min
COOKING TIME: 20 min
MODE OF COOKING: Baking
INGREDIENTS:
- 4 tilapia fillets
- 1 pint cherry tomatoes, halved
- 3 cloves garlic, minced
- 2 Tbsp olive oil
- 1/4 cup fresh basil, chopped
- Salt and pepper to taste

DIRECTIONS:
1. Preheat oven to 400°F (200°C).
2. Place tilapia fillets in a baking dish. Surround with cherry tomatoes.
3. Drizzle with olive oil and sprinkle with garlic, salt, and pepper.
4. Bake for 15-20 minutes, until fish is opaque and flakes easily with a fork.
5. Garnish with fresh basil before serving.

TIPS:
- Serve with a side of quinoa or brown rice.
- Add a splash of balsamic vinegar before baking for extra flavor.

NUTRITIONAL VALUES: Calories: 220, Fat: 10g, Carbs: 5g, Protein: 28g, Sugar: 3g

GRILLED MAHI MAHI WITH PINEAPPLE SALSA

PREPARATION TIME: 15 min
COOKING TIME: 10 min
MODE OF COOKING: Grilling
INGREDIENTS:
- 4 mahi mahi fillets
- 1 Tbsp olive oil
- 1 tsp paprika
- 1 tsp garlic powder
- 1/2 tsp salt
- 1/4 tsp black pepper
- 1 cup fresh pineapple, diced
- 1/4 cup red onion, finely chopped
- 1 jalapeño, seeded and minced
- Juice of 1 lime
- 2 Tbsp fresh cilantro, chopped

DIRECTIONS:
1. Preheat grill to medium-high heat.
2. In a small bowl, mix olive oil, paprika, garlic powder, salt, and pepper. Brush mixture over mahi mahi fillets.
3. Grill fillets for 4-5 minutes per side, until fully cooked.
4. In a separate bowl, combine pineapple, red onion, jalapeño, lime juice, and cilantro to make the salsa.
5. Serve mahi mahi topped with pineapple salsa.

TIPS:
- Serve with a side of grilled vegetables.
- Add avocado to the salsa for extra creaminess.

NUTRITIONAL VALUES: Calories: 240, Fat: 8g, Carbs: 12g, Protein: 30g, Sugar: 8g

Seared Scallops with Lemon Garlic Butter

PREPARATION TIME: 5 min
COOKING TIME: 10 min
MODE OF COOKING: Searing
INGREDIENTS:

- 1 lb sea scallops
- 2 Tbsp butter
- 3 cloves garlic, minced
- Juice of 1 lemon
- 1 Tbsp fresh parsley, chopped
- Salt and pepper to taste

DIRECTIONS:

1. Pat scallops dry with paper towels and season with salt and pepper.
2. Heat butter in a large skillet over medium-high heat.
3. Add scallops and sear for 2-3 minutes per side, until golden brown.
4. Remove scallops from the skillet and set aside.
5. In the same skillet, add garlic and cook until fragrant. Stir in lemon juice.
6. Return scallops to the skillet and toss to coat with the sauce.
7. Sprinkle with fresh parsley and serve immediately.

TIPS:

- Serve over a bed of mixed greens or alongside steamed asparagus.
- Garnish with lemon zest for extra brightness.

NUTRITIONAL VALUES: Calories: 250, Fat: 12g, Carbs: 2g, Protein: 30g, Sugar: 0g

Honey Lime Glazed Shrimp

PREPARATION TIME: 10 min
COOKING TIME: 10 min
MODE OF COOKING: Sautéing
INGREDIENTS:

- 1 lb shrimp, peeled and deveined
- 2 Tbsp olive oil
- 3 Tbsp honey
- Juice of 2 limes
- 2 cloves garlic, minced
- 1/2 tsp chili powder
- Salt and pepper to taste

DIRECTIONS:

1. In a small bowl, whisk together honey, lime juice, garlic, chili powder, salt, and pepper.
2. Heat olive oil in a large skillet over medium-high heat.
3. Add shrimp and cook until pink and opaque, about 2-3 minutes per side.
4. Pour honey lime mixture over the shrimp and toss to coat.
5. Cook for an additional 1-2 minutes, until the sauce thickens.
6. Serve immediately.

TIPS:

- Serve over cauliflower rice or mixed greens.

- Garnish with chopped cilantro and lime wedges.

NUTRITIONAL VALUES: Calories: 220, Fat: 8g, Carbs: 15g, Protein: 24g, Sugar: 12g

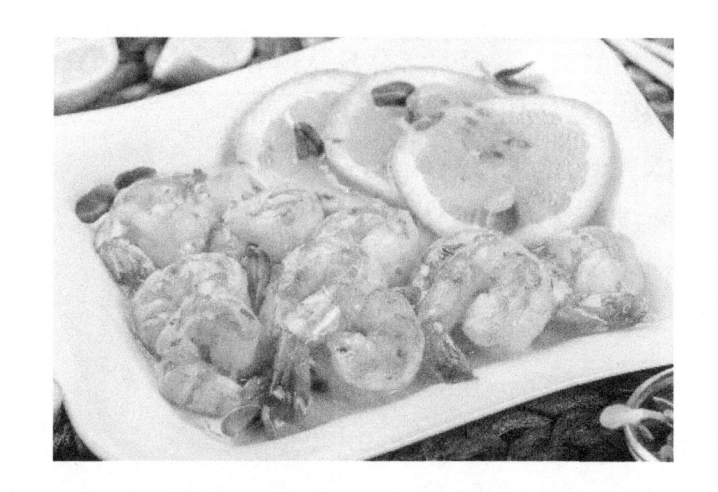

BAKED LEMON DILL HALIBUT

PREPARATION TIME: 10 min
COOKING TIME: 20 min
MODE OF COOKING: Baking
INGREDIENTS:
- 4 halibut fillets
- 2 Tbsp olive oil
- 1 lemon, sliced
- 2 Tbsp fresh dill, chopped
- Salt and pepper to taste

DIRECTIONS:
1. Preheat oven to 375°F (190°C).
2. Place halibut fillets in a baking dish. Drizzle with olive oil and season with salt and pepper.
3. Top each fillet with lemon slices and sprinkle with fresh dill.
4. Bake for 15-20 minutes, until halibut is opaque and flakes easily with a fork.
5. Serve immediately with your favorite side dish.

TIPS:
- Serve with roasted potatoes or a quinoa salad.
- Garnish with additional fresh dill before serving.

NUTRITIONAL VALUES: Calories: 270, Fat: 14g, Carbs: 2g, Protein: 34g, Sugar: 0g

CAJUN CATFISH WITH RED PEPPER AIOLI

PREPARATION TIME: 10 min
COOKING TIME: 10 min
MODE OF COOKING: Pan-Frying
INGREDIENTS:
- 4 catfish fillets
- 2 Tbsp olive oil
- 2 Tbsp Cajun seasoning
- 1/2 cup Greek yogurt
- 1/4 cup roasted red peppers, finely chopped
- 1 clove garlic, minced
- Juice of 1/2 lemon
- Salt and pepper to taste

DIRECTIONS:
1. Rub catfish fillets with Cajun seasoning on both sides.

2. Heat olive oil in a large skillet over medium-high heat.
3. Add catfish fillets and cook for 3-4 minutes per side, until golden and fully cooked.
4. In a small bowl, mix Greek yogurt, roasted red peppers, garlic, lemon juice, salt, and pepper to make the aioli.
5. Serve catfish fillets with a dollop of red pepper aioli.

TIPS:
- Serve with a side of coleslaw or grilled vegetables.
- Garnish with fresh parsley.

NUTRITIONAL VALUES: Calories: 310, Fat: 15g, Carbs: 4g, Protein: 36g, Sugar: 2g

GRILLED SWORDFISH WITH MANGO SALSA

PREPARATION TIME: 15 min
COOKING TIME: 10 min
MODE OF COOKING: Grilling
INGREDIENTS:
- 4 swordfish steaks
- 2 Tbsp olive oil
- 1 tsp paprika
- 1 tsp garlic powder
- 1/2 tsp salt
- 1/4 tsp black pepper
- 1 cup mango, diced
- 1/4 cup red onion, finely chopped
- 1 jalapeño, seeded and minced
- Juice of 1 lime
- 2 Tbsp fresh cilantro, chopped

DIRECTIONS:
1. Preheat grill to medium-high heat.
2. In a small bowl, mix olive oil, paprika, garlic powder, salt, and pepper. Brush mixture over swordfish steaks.
3. Grill steaks for 4-5 minutes per side, until fully cooked.
4. In a separate bowl, combine mango, red onion, jalapeño, lime juice, and cilantro to make the salsa.
5. Serve swordfish topped with mango salsa.

TIPS:
- Serve with a side of grilled asparagus.
- Add avocado to the salsa for extra creaminess.

NUTRITIONAL VALUES: Calories: 280, Fat: 12g, Carbs: 12g, Protein: 34g, Sugar: 8g

CHAPTER 10: POULTRY AND BEEF FAVORITES

LEMON HERB CHICKEN

PREPARATION TIME: 10 min
COOKING TIME: 30 min
MODE OF COOKING: Baking
INGREDIENTS:

- 4 boneless, skinless chicken breasts
- 2 Tbsp olive oil
- 2 cloves garlic, minced
- Juice and zest of 1 lemon
- 1 tsp dried oregano
- 1 tsp dried thyme
- Salt and pepper to taste

DIRECTIONS:

1. Preheat oven to 375°F (190°C).
2. In a small bowl, whisk together olive oil, garlic, lemon juice, lemon zest, oregano, thyme, salt, and pepper.
3. Place chicken breasts in a baking dish and brush with the lemon herb mixture.
4. Bake for 25-30 minutes, or until chicken is fully cooked and juices run clear.
5. Serve immediately with your favorite side dish.

TIPS:

- Serve with roasted vegetables or a fresh salad.
- Garnish with fresh parsley for extra color.

NUTRITIONAL VALUES: Calories: 280, Fat: 12g, Carbs: 2g, Protein: 40g, Sugar: 0g

BALSAMIC GLAZED STEAK

PREPARATION TIME: 10 min
COOKING TIME: 15 min
MODE OF COOKING: Grilling
INGREDIENTS:

- 4 beef steaks (sirloin, ribeye, or your choice)
- 1/4 cup balsamic vinegar
- 2 Tbsp olive oil
- 2 cloves garlic, minced
- 1 Tbsp honey
- Salt and pepper to taste

DIRECTIONS:

1. In a small bowl, whisk together balsamic vinegar, olive oil, garlic, honey, salt, and pepper.
2. Marinate the steaks in the balsamic mixture for at least 30 minutes.
3. Preheat grill to medium-high heat.
4. Grill steaks for 5-7 minutes per side, or until desired doneness.
5. Let steaks rest for 5 minutes before serving.

TIPS:

- Serve with grilled asparagus or a side of mashed cauliflower.
- Top with fresh herbs like rosemary or thyme for added flavor.

NUTRITIONAL VALUES: Calories: 350, Fat: 20g, Carbs: 5g, Protein: 35g, Sugar: 4g

GARLIC ROSEMARY ROAST CHICKEN

PREPARATION TIME: 15 min
COOKING TIME: 1 hr 20 min
MODE OF COOKING: Roasting
INGREDIENTS:
- 1 whole chicken (about 4 lbs)
- 3 Tbsp olive oil
- 4 cloves garlic, minced
- 2 Tbsp fresh rosemary, chopped
- Juice of 1 lemon
- Salt and pepper to taste

DIRECTIONS:
1. Preheat oven to 375°F (190°C).
2. In a small bowl, mix olive oil, garlic, rosemary, lemon juice, salt, and pepper.
3. Rub the mixture all over the chicken, including under the skin.
4. Place chicken in a roasting pan and roast for 1 hour and 20 minutes, or until internal temperature reaches 165°F (74°C).
5. Let rest for 10 minutes before carving and serving.

TIPS:
- Serve with roasted root vegetables.
- Use the pan drippings to make a flavorful gravy.

NUTRITIONAL VALUES: Calories: 400, Fat: 25g, Carbs: 3g, Protein: 38g, Sugar: 0g

TERIYAKI BEEF STIR-FRY

PREPARATION TIME: 10 min
COOKING TIME: 15 min
MODE OF COOKING: Stir-Frying
INGREDIENTS:
- 1 lb beef sirloin, thinly sliced
- 2 Tbsp olive oil
- 1 red bell pepper, sliced
- 1 green bell pepper, sliced
- 1 yellow onion, sliced
- 1/4 cup soy sauce
- 2 Tbsp honey
- 1 Tbsp rice vinegar
- 2 cloves garlic, minced
- 1 tsp grated ginger
- 1 tsp cornstarch
- 1/4 cup water

DIRECTIONS:
1. In a small bowl, mix soy sauce, honey, rice vinegar, garlic, ginger, cornstarch, and water.
2. Heat olive oil in a large skillet or wok over medium-high heat.
3. Add beef and stir-fry until browned, about 3-4 minutes.
4. Add bell peppers and onion, stir-fry for another 5 minutes.

5. Pour the sauce over the beef and vegetables, stir well and cook for another 2-3 minutes until the sauce thickens.
6. Serve immediately.

TIPS:
- Serve over cauliflower rice or steamed broccoli.
- Garnish with sesame seeds and green onions.

NUTRITIONAL VALUES: Calories: 300, Fat: 15g, Carbs: 12g, Protein: 28g, Sugar: 8g

HERB-CRUSTED PORK TENDERLOIN

PREPARATION TIME: 15 min
COOKING TIME: 25 min
MODE OF COOKING: Roasting
INGREDIENTS:
- 1 pork tenderloin (about 1 lb)
- 2 Tbsp olive oil
- 1 Tbsp Dijon mustard
- 2 cloves garlic, minced
- 1 tsp dried thyme
- 1 tsp dried rosemary
- Salt and pepper to taste

DIRECTIONS:
1. Preheat oven to 400°F (200°C).
2. In a small bowl, mix olive oil, Dijon mustard, garlic, thyme, rosemary, salt, and pepper.
3. Rub the mixture all over the pork tenderloin.
4. Place tenderloin on a baking sheet and roast for 25 minutes, or until internal temperature reaches 145°F (63°C).
5. Let rest for 5 minutes before slicing and serving.

TIPS:
- Serve with roasted Brussels sprouts or a green salad.
- Use leftover pork in sandwiches or salads.

NUTRITIONAL VALUES: Calories: 280, Fat: 12g, Carbs: 2g, Protein: 40g, Sugar: 0g

SPICY CHICKEN SKEWERS

PREPARATION TIME: 15 min
COOKING TIME: 10 min
MODE OF COOKING: Grilling
INGREDIENTS:
- 2 boneless, skinless chicken breasts, cut into cubes
- 2 Tbsp olive oil
- 1 tsp paprika
- 1/2 tsp cayenne pepper
- 1 tsp garlic powder
- 1 tsp onion powder
- Salt and pepper to taste
- Wooden skewers, soaked in water

DIRECTIONS:
1. Preheat grill to medium-high heat.
2. In a large bowl, mix olive oil, paprika, cayenne pepper, garlic powder, onion powder, salt, and pepper.
3. Add chicken cubes to the bowl and toss to coat evenly.
4. Thread chicken onto wooden skewers.
5. Grill skewers for 5-6 minutes per side, or until fully cooked.
6. Serve immediately.

TIPS:
- Serve with a side of tzatziki or a fresh cucumber salad.
- Garnish with chopped fresh cilantro.

NUTRITIONAL VALUES: Calories: 220, Fat: 10g, Carbs: 2g, Protein: 28g, Sugar: 0g

Lemon Basil Chicken

PREPARATION TIME: 10 min
COOKING TIME: 20 min
MODE OF COOKING: Sautéing
INGREDIENTS:
- 4 boneless, skinless chicken breasts
- 2 Tbsp olive oil
- 1/2 cup chicken broth
- Juice and zest of 1 lemon
- 1/4 cup fresh basil, chopped
- 2 cloves garlic, minced
- Salt and pepper to taste

DIRECTIONS:
1. Heat olive oil in a large skillet over medium-high heat.
2. Season chicken breasts with salt and pepper and add to the skillet.
3. Cook for 5-7 minutes per side, until golden brown and cooked through.
4. Remove chicken from the skillet and set aside.
5. In the same skillet, add garlic and sauté until fragrant.
6. Add chicken broth, lemon juice, and lemon zest, and bring to a simmer.
7. Return chicken to the skillet and cook for another 2-3 minutes, until heated through.
8. Stir in fresh basil before serving.

TIPS:
- Serve with a side of steamed vegetables or quinoa.
- Garnish with extra lemon zest and basil.

NUTRITIONAL VALUES: Calories: 250, Fat: 10g, Carbs: 2g, Protein: 36g, Sugar: 0g

Herb-Marinated Flank Steak

PREPARATION TIME: 10 min
COOKING TIME: 15 min
MODE OF COOKING: Grilling
INGREDIENTS:
- 1 1/2 lbs flank steak
- 1/4 cup olive oil

- 2 Tbsp red wine vinegar
- 2 cloves garlic, minced
- 1 Tbsp fresh rosemary, chopped
- 1 Tbsp fresh thyme, chopped
- Salt and pepper to taste

DIRECTIONS:

1. In a small bowl, whisk together olive oil, red wine vinegar, garlic, rosemary, thyme, salt, and pepper.
2. Place flank steak in a large resealable bag and pour marinade over the steak. Marinate for at least 30 minutes.
3. Preheat grill to medium-high heat.
4. Grill steak for 6-8 minutes per side, or until desired doneness.
5. Let steak rest for 5 minutes before slicing against the grain.
6. Serve immediately.

TIPS:

- Serve with a side of grilled vegetables or a fresh salad.
- Garnish with extra fresh herbs.

NUTRITIONAL VALUES: Calories: 320, Fat: 18g, Carbs: 2g, Protein: 36g, Sugar: 0g

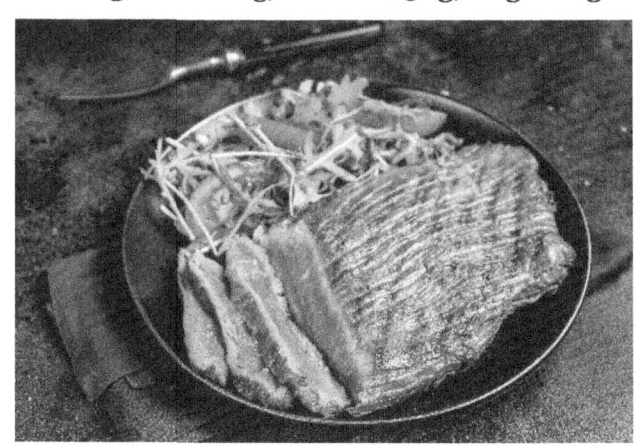

BBQ Chicken Thighs

PREPARATION TIME: 10 min
COOKING TIME: 40 min
MODE OF COOKING: Baking
INGREDIENTS:

- 8 chicken thighs, bone-in, skin-on
- 1/2 cup BBQ sauce
- 2 Tbsp olive oil
- 2 cloves garlic, minced
- 1 tsp smoked paprika
- Salt and pepper to taste

DIRECTIONS:

1. Preheat oven to 375°F (190°C).
2. In a small bowl, mix BBQ sauce, olive oil, garlic, smoked paprika, salt, and pepper.
3. Place chicken thighs in a baking dish and brush with the BBQ sauce mixture.
4. Bake for 35-40 minutes, or until chicken is fully cooked and skin is crispy.
5. Serve immediately.

TIPS:

- Serve with coleslaw or roasted sweet potatoes.
- Brush with extra BBQ sauce before serving for more flavor.

NUTRITIONAL VALUES: Calories: 380, Fat: 25g, Carbs: 6g, Protein: 30g, Sugar: 4g

CHAPTER 11: FRESH AND FLAVORFUL SALADS

GRILLED CHICKEN CAESAR SALAD

PREPARATION TIME: 15 min
COOKING TIME: 10 min
MODE OF COOKING: Grilling
INGREDIENTS:
- 2 boneless, skinless chicken breasts
- 1 Tbsp olive oil
- Salt and pepper to taste
- 4 cups romaine lettuce, chopped
- 1/4 cup grated Parmesan cheese
- 1/2 cup Caesar dressing
- 1/4 cup croutons (optional)

DIRECTIONS:
1. Preheat grill to medium-high heat.
2. Brush chicken breasts with olive oil and season with salt and pepper.
3. Grill chicken for 5-6 minutes per side, until fully cooked. Let rest for 5 minutes before slicing.
4. In a large bowl, combine romaine lettuce, Parmesan cheese, Caesar dressing, and croutons if using.
5. Top with sliced grilled chicken and serve immediately.

TIPS:
- Use a homemade Caesar dressing for a fresher taste.
- Add a squeeze of lemon juice for extra zing.

NUTRITIONAL VALUES: Calories: 350, Fat: 24g, Carbs: 6g, Protein: 25g, Sugar: 2g

GREEK SALAD WITH GRILLED SHRIMP

PREPARATION TIME: 15 min
COOKING TIME: 10 min
MODE OF COOKING: Grilling
INGREDIENTS:
- 1 lb shrimp, peeled and deveined
- 2 Tbsp olive oil
- 1 tsp dried oregano
- Salt and pepper to taste
- 4 cups mixed greens
- 1 cup cherry tomatoes, halved
- 1 cucumber, sliced
- 1/4 cup red onion, thinly sliced
- 1/4 cup Kalamata olives
- 1/4 cup feta cheese, crumbled
- 1/4 cup Greek dressing

DIRECTIONS:
1. Preheat grill to medium-high heat.
2. Toss shrimp with olive oil, dried oregano, salt, and pepper.
3. Grill shrimp for 2-3 minutes per side, until pink and opaque.
4. In a large bowl, combine mixed greens, cherry tomatoes, cucumber, red onion, Kalamata olives, and feta cheese.
5. Top with grilled shrimp and drizzle with Greek dressing before serving.

TIPS:
- Add a sprinkle of fresh dill for extra flavor.
- Serve with whole grain pita bread.

NUTRITIONAL VALUES: Calories: 300, Fat: 20g, Carbs: 8g, Protein: 20g, Sugar: 4g

AVOCADO AND MANGO SALAD

PREPARATION TIME: 10 min
COOKING TIME: 0 min
MODE OF COOKING: Assembling
INGREDIENTS:
- 2 ripe avocados, diced
- 1 ripe mango, diced
- 1/4 cup red onion, finely chopped
- 1/4 cup fresh cilantro, chopped
- Juice of 1 lime
- Salt and pepper to taste

DIRECTIONS:
1. In a large bowl, combine diced avocado, mango, red onion, and cilantro.
2. Drizzle with lime juice and season with salt and pepper.
3. Toss gently to combine and serve immediately.

TIPS:
- Add a dash of cayenne pepper for a spicy kick.
- Serve as a side dish with grilled fish or chicken.

NUTRITIONAL VALUES: Calories: 200, Fat: 14g, Carbs: 21g, Protein: 2g, Sugar: 10g

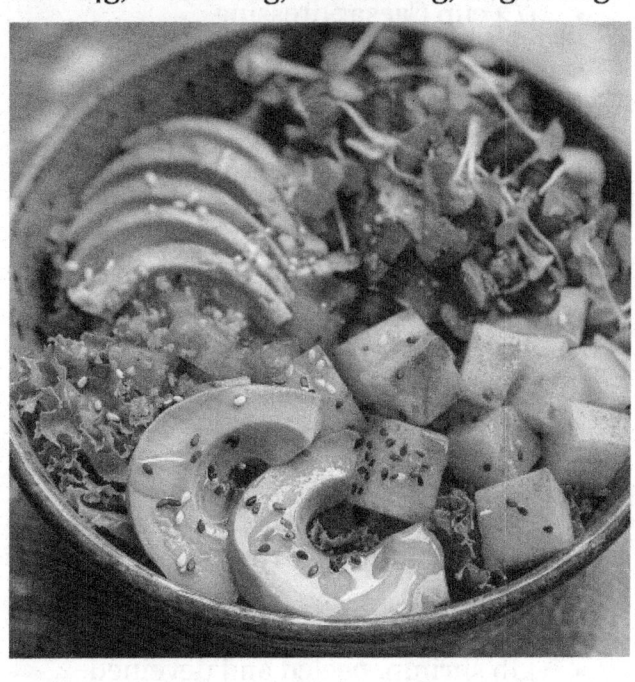

SPINACH AND STRAWBERRY SALAD

PREPARATION TIME: 10 min
COOKING TIME: 0 min
MODE OF COOKING: Assembling
INGREDIENTS:
- 4 cups fresh spinach
- 1 cup strawberries, sliced
- 1/4 cup red onion, thinly sliced
- 1/4 cup feta cheese, crumbled
- 1/4 cup sliced almonds, toasted
- 1/4 cup balsamic vinaigrette

DIRECTIONS:
1. In a large bowl, combine spinach, strawberries, red onion, feta cheese, and sliced almonds.
2. Drizzle with balsamic vinaigrette and toss gently to combine.

3. Serve immediately.

TIPS:
- Add grilled chicken for a complete meal.
- Use a raspberry vinaigrette for a different flavor.

NUTRITIONAL VALUES: Calories: 220, Fat: 14g, Carbs: 18g, Protein: 6g, Sugar: 8g

QUINOA AND BLACK BEAN SALAD

PREPARATION TIME: 15 min
COOKING TIME: 15 min
MODE OF COOKING: Boiling
INGREDIENTS:
- 1 cup quinoa, rinsed
- 2 cups water
- 1 can black beans, rinsed and drained
- 1 cup cherry tomatoes, halved
- 1/2 cup corn kernels
- 1/4 cup red onion, finely chopped
- 1/4 cup fresh cilantro, chopped
- 1/4 cup lime juice
- 2 Tbsp olive oil
- Salt and pepper to taste

DIRECTIONS:
1. In a medium saucepan, bring quinoa and water to a boil. Reduce heat, cover, and simmer for 15 minutes or until water is absorbed. Let cool.
2. In a large bowl, combine cooked quinoa, black beans, cherry tomatoes, corn, red onion, and cilantro.
3. In a small bowl, whisk together lime juice, olive oil, salt, and pepper. Pour over salad and toss to combine.
4. Serve immediately or chill in the refrigerator before serving.

TIPS:
- Add diced avocado for extra creaminess.
- Serve with tortilla chips for added crunch.

NUTRITIONAL VALUES: Calories: 250, Fat: 8g, Carbs: 36g, Protein: 9g, Sugar: 3g

CHICKEN AND AVOCADO SALAD

PREPARATION TIME: 15 min
COOKING TIME: 0 min
MODE OF COOKING: Assembling
INGREDIENTS:
- 2 cups cooked chicken breast, shredded
- 1 ripe avocado, diced
- 1/4 cup red onion, finely chopped
- 1/4 cup celery, diced
- 2 Tbsp fresh cilantro, chopped
- 1/4 cup Greek yogurt
- 1 Tbsp lime juice
- Salt and pepper to taste

DIRECTIONS:
1. In a large bowl, combine shredded chicken, avocado, red onion, celery, and cilantro.
2. In a small bowl, mix Greek yogurt,

lime juice, salt, and pepper. Pour over the chicken mixture and toss gently to combine.

3. Serve immediately or chill in the refrigerator before serving.

TIPS:
- Serve in lettuce wraps for a low-carb option.
- Add a pinch of smoked paprika for extra flavor.

NUTRITIONAL VALUES: Calories: 280, Fat: 16g, Carbs: 8g, Protein: 24g, Sugar: 2g

CAPRESE SALAD

PREPARATION TIME: 10 min
COOKING TIME: 0 min
MODE OF COOKING: Assembling
INGREDIENTS:
- 4 ripe tomatoes, sliced
- 1 lb fresh mozzarella, sliced
- 1/4 cup fresh basil leaves
- 2 Tbsp balsamic glaze
- 2 Tbsp olive oil
- Salt and pepper to taste

DIRECTIONS:
1. Arrange tomato and mozzarella slices on a platter, alternating between the two.
2. Tuck basil leaves between the slices.
3. Drizzle with balsamic glaze and olive oil.
4. Season with salt and pepper and serve immediately.

TIPS:
- Use heirloom tomatoes for a more colorful presentation.
- Add a sprinkle of crushed red pepper for a hint of spice.

NUTRITIONAL VALUES: Calories: 200, Fat: 16g, Carbs: 6g, Protein: 10g, Sugar: 3g

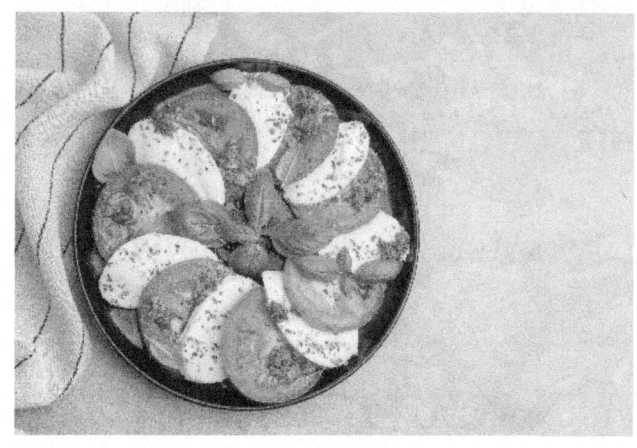

MEDITERRANEAN CHICKPEA SALAD

PREPARATION TIME: 10 min
COOKING TIME: 0 min
MODE OF COOKING: Assembling
INGREDIENTS:
- 1 can chickpeas, rinsed and drained
- 1 cup cherry tomatoes, halved
- 1 cucumber, diced
- 1/4 cup red onion, finely chopped
- 1/4 cup Kalamata olives, sliced
- 1/4 cup feta cheese, crumbled
- 2 Tbsp olive oil
- 1 Tbsp red wine vinegar

- 1 tsp dried oregano
- Salt and pepper to taste

DIRECTIONS:
1. In a large bowl, combine chickpeas, cherry tomatoes, cucumber, red onion, Kalamata olives, and feta cheese.
2. In a small bowl, whisk together olive oil, red wine vinegar, oregano, salt, and pepper. Pour over the salad and toss gently to combine.
3. Serve immediately or chill in the refrigerator before serving.

TIPS:
- Add fresh parsley for extra flavor.
- Serve with whole grain pita bread.

NUTRITIONAL VALUES: Calories: 220, Fat: 12g, Carbs: 20g, Protein: 8g, Sugar: 4g

ASIAN CHICKEN SALAD

PREPARATION TIME: 15 min
COOKING TIME: 10 min
MODE OF COOKING: Grilling
INGREDIENTS:
- 2 boneless, skinless chicken breasts
- 2 Tbsp soy sauce
- 1 Tbsp honey
- 1 Tbsp rice vinegar
- 1 tsp sesame oil
- 4 cups mixed greens
- 1 cup shredded cabbage
- 1/2 cup shredded carrots
- 1/4 cup sliced almonds
- 2 green onions, sliced
- 1/4 cup sesame ginger dressing

DIRECTIONS:
1. In a small bowl, whisk together soy sauce, honey, rice vinegar, and sesame oil. Marinate chicken breasts in the mixture for at least 30 minutes.
2. Preheat grill to medium-high heat.
3. Grill chicken for 5-6 minutes per side, until fully cooked. Let rest for 5 minutes before slicing.
4. In a large bowl, combine mixed greens, shredded cabbage, shredded carrots, sliced almonds, and green onions.
5. Top with sliced grilled chicken and drizzle with sesame ginger dressing before serving.

TIPS:
- Add a sprinkle of sesame seeds for extra texture.
- Serve with a side of edamame.

NUTRITIONAL VALUES: Calories: 350, Fat: 20g, Carbs: 15g, Protein: 30g, Sugar: 8g

Avocado and Tuna Salad

PREPARATION TIME: 10 min
COOKING TIME: 0 min
MODE OF COOKING: Assembling
INGREDIENTS:

- 2 cans tuna, drained
- 1 ripe avocado, diced
- 1/4 cup red onion, finely chopped
- 1/4 cup celery, diced
- 2 Tbsp fresh parsley, chopped
- 1/4 cup Greek yogurt
- Juice of 1 lemon
- Salt and pepper to taste

DIRECTIONS:

1. In a large bowl, combine drained tuna, diced avocado, red onion, celery, and parsley.
2. In a small bowl, mix Greek yogurt, lemon juice, salt, and pepper. Pour over the tuna mixture and toss gently to combine.
3. Serve immediately or chill in the refrigerator before serving.

TIPS:

- Serve in lettuce wraps for a low-carb option.
- Add a pinch of cayenne pepper for a spicy kick.

NUTRITIONAL VALUES: Calories: 250, Fat: 14g, Carbs: 6g, Protein: 24g, Sugar: 2g

CHAPTER 12: DELICIOUS VEGETARIAN OPTIONS

QUINOA STUFFED BELL PEPPERS

PREPARATION TIME: 15 min
COOKING TIME: 30 min
MODE OF COOKING: Baking
INGREDIENTS:

- 4 bell peppers, halved and seeded
- 1 cup quinoa, rinsed
- 2 cups vegetable broth
- 1 cup black beans, rinsed and drained
- 1 cup corn kernels
- 1 cup diced tomatoes
- 1/4 cup red onion, finely chopped
- 2 cloves garlic, minced
- 1 tsp cumin
- 1 tsp chili powder
- Salt and pepper to taste
- 1/4 cup fresh cilantro, chopped

DIRECTIONS:

1. Preheat oven to 375°F (190°C).
2. In a medium saucepan, bring quinoa and vegetable broth to a boil. Reduce heat, cover, and simmer for 15 minutes or until liquid is absorbed.
3. In a large bowl, combine cooked quinoa, black beans, corn, diced tomatoes, red onion, garlic, cumin, chili powder, salt, and pepper.
4. Stuff each bell pepper half with the quinoa mixture and place in a baking dish.
5. Cover with foil and bake for 25 minutes. Remove foil and bake for an additional 5 minutes.
6. Garnish with fresh cilantro before serving.

TIPS:

- Add a sprinkle of cheese on top before the final 5 minutes of baking.
- Serve with a side of guacamole or salsa.

NUTRITIONAL VALUES: Calories: 250, Fat: 5g, Carbs: 45g, Protein: 10g, Sugar: 8g

LENTIL AND SWEET POTATO STEW

PREPARATION TIME: 15 min
COOKING TIME: 40 min
MODE OF COOKING: Simmering
INGREDIENTS:

- 1 cup green lentils, rinsed
- 2 medium sweet potatoes, peeled and diced
- 1 can diced tomatoes
- 1 onion, chopped
- 3 cloves garlic, minced
- 1 tsp cumin
- 1 tsp smoked paprika
- 4 cups vegetable broth
- 2 cups kale, chopped
- 2 Tbsp olive oil
- Salt and pepper to taste

DIRECTIONS:

1. In a large pot, heat olive oil over

medium heat. Add onion and garlic, sauté until softened.
2. Stir in cumin and smoked paprika, cooking for another minute.
3. Add lentils, sweet potatoes, diced tomatoes, and vegetable broth. Bring to a boil.
4. Reduce heat and simmer for 30 minutes, or until lentils and sweet potatoes are tender.
5. Stir in chopped kale and cook for an additional 5 minutes.
6. Season with salt and pepper to taste and serve hot.

TIPS:
- Serve with crusty bread for a hearty meal.
- Add a splash of apple cider vinegar for a tangy twist.

NUTRITIONAL VALUES: Calories: 300, Fat: 8g, Carbs: 50g, Protein: 12g, Sugar: 8g

CHICKPEA AND SPINACH CURRY

PREPARATION TIME: 10 min
COOKING TIME: 20 min
MODE OF COOKING: Simmering
INGREDIENTS:
- 1 can chickpeas, rinsed and drained
- 4 cups fresh spinach
- 1 onion, finely chopped
- 3 cloves garlic, minced
- 1 Tbsp ginger, minced
- 1 can coconut milk
- 1 can diced tomatoes
- 1 Tbsp curry powder
- 1 tsp turmeric
- 2 Tbsp olive oil
- Salt and pepper to taste

DIRECTIONS:
1. In a large skillet, heat olive oil over medium heat. Add onion, garlic, and ginger, sauté until softened.
2. Stir in curry powder and turmeric, cooking for another minute.
3. Add chickpeas, coconut milk, and diced tomatoes. Bring to a simmer.
4. Stir in fresh spinach and cook until wilted.
5. Season with salt and pepper to taste and serve hot.

TIPS:
- Serve over basmati rice or quinoa.
- Garnish with fresh cilantro and a squeeze of lime.

NUTRITIONAL VALUES: Calories: 280, Fat: 15g, Carbs: 30g, Protein: 9g, Sugar: 6g

ROASTED VEGETABLE AND HUMMUS WRAP

PREPARATION TIME: 15 min
COOKING TIME: 25 min
MODE OF COOKING: Roasting

INGREDIENTS:
- 1 zucchini, sliced
- 1 red bell pepper, sliced
- 1 yellow bell pepper, sliced
- 1 red onion, sliced
- 2 Tbsp olive oil
- Salt and pepper to taste
- 1 cup hummus
- 4 whole wheat tortillas
- 1/4 cup fresh basil, chopped

DIRECTIONS:
1. Preheat oven to 400°F (200°C).
2. Place zucchini, red bell pepper, yellow bell pepper, and red onion on a baking sheet. Drizzle with olive oil, and season with salt and pepper.
3. Roast for 20-25 minutes, or until vegetables are tender and lightly browned.
4. Spread hummus evenly on each tortilla.
5. Top with roasted vegetables and sprinkle with fresh basil.
6. Roll up each tortilla and serve immediately.

TIPS:
- Add a drizzle of balsamic glaze for extra flavor.
- Serve with a side salad for a complete meal.

NUTRITIONAL VALUES: Calories: 350, Fat: 14g, Carbs: 45g, Protein: 10g, Sugar: 6g

SPAGHETTI SQUASH WITH MARINARA SAUCE

PREPARATION TIME: 10 min
COOKING TIME: 40 min
MODE OF COOKING: Baking and Simmering

INGREDIENTS:
- 1 large spaghetti squash
- 2 cups marinara sauce
- 1/4 cup Parmesan cheese, grated
- 2 Tbsp olive oil
- 1 tsp dried basil
- 1 tsp dried oregano
- Salt and pepper to taste

DIRECTIONS:
1. Preheat oven to 400°F (200°C).
2. Cut the spaghetti squash in half lengthwise and scoop out seeds.
3. Brush the inside with olive oil, and season with salt and pepper.
4. Place squash halves cut-side down on a baking sheet and bake for 35-40 minutes, or until tender.
5. In a medium saucepan, heat marinara sauce over medium heat. Stir in dried basil and oregano.
6. Use a fork to scrape the flesh of the spaghetti squash into strands.
7. Top with marinara sauce and grated Parmesan cheese before serving.

TIPS:
- Add sautéed mushrooms or spinach to the marinara sauce for extra veggies.
- Serve with a side of garlic bread.

NUTRITIONAL VALUES: Calories: 250, Fat: 10g, Carbs: 35g, Protein: 7g, Sugar: 12g

GRILLED PORTOBELLO MUSHROOMS

PREPARATION TIME: 10 min
COOKING TIME: 10 min
MODE OF COOKING: Grilling
INGREDIENTS:

- 4 large portobello mushrooms
- 3 Tbsp balsamic vinegar
- 2 Tbsp olive oil
- 2 cloves garlic, minced
- Salt and pepper to taste

DIRECTIONS:

1. In a small bowl, whisk together balsamic vinegar, olive oil, garlic, salt, and pepper.
2. Brush the mixture onto both sides of the portobello mushrooms.
3. Preheat grill to medium-high heat.
4. Grill mushrooms for 4-5 minutes per side, or until tender and juicy.
5. Serve immediately.

TIPS:

- Serve as a burger replacement with your favorite toppings.
- Garnish with fresh herbs like parsley or basil.

NUTRITIONAL VALUES: Calories: 120, Fat: 10g, Carbs: 7g, Protein: 2g, Sugar: 3g

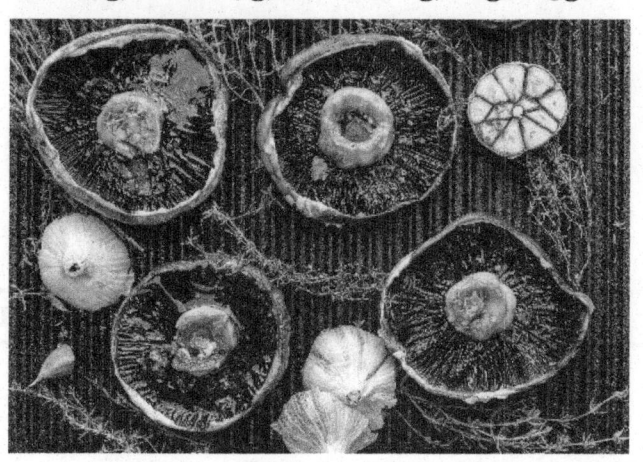

VEGAN STUFFED ZUCCHINI BOATS

PREPARATION TIME: 15 min
COOKING TIME: 30 min
MODE OF COOKING: Baking
INGREDIENTS:

- 4 medium zucchinis, halved lengthwise and seeded
- 1 cup cooked quinoa
- 1 cup black beans, rinsed and drained
- 1 cup corn kernels
- 1/2 cup salsa
- 1/4 cup fresh cilantro, chopped
- 1 tsp cumin
- Salt and pepper to taste

DIRECTIONS:

1. Preheat oven to 375°F (190°C).
2. In a large bowl, combine cooked quinoa, black beans, corn, salsa, cilantro, cumin, salt, and pepper.
3. Stuff each zucchini half with the quinoa mixture and place in a baking

dish.
4. Cover with foil and bake for 25 minutes. Remove foil and bake for an additional 5 minutes.
5. Serve immediately.

TIPS:
- Top with avocado slices or a dollop of guacamole.
- Add a sprinkle of vegan cheese before baking.

NUTRITIONAL VALUES: Calories: 200, Fat: 4g, Carbs: 35g, Protein: 7g, Sugar: 6g

EGGPLANT PARMESAN

PREPARATION TIME: 15 min
COOKING TIME: 45 min
MODE OF COOKING: Baking
INGREDIENTS:
- 2 large eggplants, sliced into rounds
- 1 cup marinara sauce
- 1 cup mozzarella cheese, shredded
- 1/4 cup Parmesan cheese, grated
- 2 Tbsp olive oil
- 1 tsp dried basil
- 1 tsp dried oregano
- Salt and pepper to taste

DIRECTIONS:
1. Preheat oven to 375°F (190°C).
2. Brush eggplant slices with olive oil and season with salt and pepper. Place on a baking sheet and bake for 20 minutes, flipping halfway through.
3. In a baking dish, layer eggplant slices, marinara sauce, mozzarella cheese, and Parmesan cheese. Repeat layers until all ingredients are used.
4. Sprinkle dried basil and oregano on top.
5. Bake for 25 minutes, or until cheese is bubbly and golden.
6. Serve immediately.

TIPS:
- Serve with a side of pasta or a green salad.
- Garnish with fresh basil before serving.

NUTRITIONAL VALUES: Calories: 300, Fat: 18g, Carbs: 24g, Protein: 12g, Sugar: 10g

CAULIFLOWER FRIED RICE

PREPARATION TIME: 10 min
COOKING TIME: 15 min
MODE OF COOKING: Sautéing
INGREDIENTS:
- 1 head cauliflower, grated into rice-sized pieces
- 1 cup mixed vegetables (peas, carrots, bell peppers)
- 2 cloves garlic, minced
- 2 Tbsp soy sauce

- 2 Tbsp sesame oil
- 2 green onions, sliced
- 1 Tbsp fresh ginger, minced
- Salt and pepper to taste

DIRECTIONS:
1. In a large skillet, heat sesame oil over medium-high heat. Add garlic and ginger, sauté until fragrant.
2. Add mixed vegetables and cook for 5 minutes, until tender.
3. Stir in cauliflower rice and soy sauce. Cook for another 5-7 minutes, until cauliflower is tender.
4. Season with salt and pepper to taste and garnish with green onions before serving.

TIPS:
- Add a scrambled egg for extra protein.
- Serve with a side of tofu or tempeh.

NUTRITIONAL VALUES: Calories: 150, Fat: 10g, Carbs: 12g, Protein: 4g, Sugar: 4g

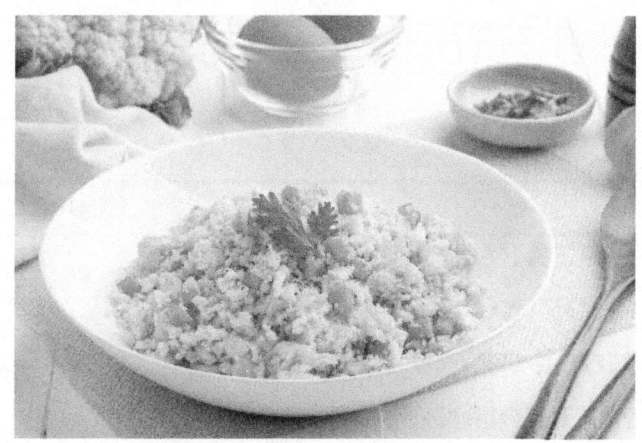

SPINACH AND RICOTTA STUFFED SHELLS

PREPARATION TIME: 20 min
COOKING TIME: 30 min
MODE OF COOKING: Baking
INGREDIENTS:
- 12 jumbo pasta shells
- 1 cup ricotta cheese
- 2 cups fresh spinach, chopped
- 1/4 cup Parmesan cheese, grated
- 1 egg, beaten
- 1 cup marinara sauce
- 1/2 cup mozzarella cheese, shredded
- Salt and pepper to taste

DIRECTIONS:
1. Preheat oven to 375°F (190°C).
2. Cook pasta shells according to package instructions. Drain and set aside.
3. In a large bowl, combine ricotta cheese, spinach, Parmesan cheese, egg, salt, and pepper.
4. Stuff each pasta shell with the ricotta mixture and place in a baking dish.
5. Pour marinara sauce over the stuffed shells and top with mozzarella cheese.
6. Cover with foil and bake for 20 minutes. Remove foil and bake for an additional 10 minutes, or until cheese is bubbly and golden.
7. Serve immediately.

TIPS:
- Garnish with fresh basil or parsley.
- Serve with a side of garlic bread.

NUTRITIONAL VALUES: Calories: 320, Fat: 16g, Carbs: 30g, Protein: 15g, Sugar: 6g

CHAPTER 13: HEARTY SOUPS AND STEWS

TUSCAN WHITE BEAN SOUP

PREPARATION TIME: 15 min
COOKING TIME: 30 min
MODE OF COOKING: Simmering
INGREDIENTS:
- 1 Tbsp olive oil
- 1 onion, diced
- 2 cloves garlic, minced
- 2 carrots, diced
- 2 celery stalks, diced
- 1 can diced tomatoes
- 4 cups vegetable broth
- 2 cans cannellini beans, rinsed and drained
- 2 cups kale, chopped
- 1 tsp dried thyme
- 1 tsp dried rosemary
- Salt and pepper to taste

DIRECTIONS:
1. In a large pot, heat olive oil over medium heat. Add onion and garlic, sauté until softened.
2. Add carrots and celery, cook for 5 minutes.
3. Stir in diced tomatoes, vegetable broth, cannellini beans, thyme, rosemary, salt, and pepper. Bring to a boil.
4. Reduce heat and simmer for 20 minutes.
5. Stir in chopped kale and cook for an additional 5 minutes.
6. Serve hot.

TIPS:
- Serve with crusty bread for a complete meal.
- Add a sprinkle of Parmesan cheese for extra flavor.

NUTRITIONAL VALUES: Calories: 250, Fat: 5g, Carbs: 40g, Protein: 12g, Sugar: 6g

SPICY LENTIL STEW

PREPARATION TIME: 10 min
COOKING TIME: 40 min
MODE OF COOKING: Simmering
INGREDIENTS:
- 1 Tbsp olive oil
- 1 onion, diced
- 2 cloves garlic, minced
- 1 tsp ginger, minced
- 2 carrots, diced
- 1 red bell pepper, diced
- 1 cup red lentils, rinsed
- 4 cups vegetable broth
- 1 can diced tomatoes
- 1 tsp cumin
- 1 tsp turmeric
- 1/2 tsp cayenne pepper
- Salt and pepper to taste
- 2 cups spinach, chopped

DIRECTIONS:

1. In a large pot, heat olive oil over medium heat. Add onion, garlic, and ginger, sauté until softened.
2. Add carrots and red bell pepper, cook for 5 minutes.
3. Stir in red lentils, vegetable broth, diced tomatoes, cumin, turmeric, cayenne pepper, salt, and pepper. Bring to a boil.
4. Reduce heat and simmer for 30 minutes, until lentils are tender.
5. Stir in chopped spinach and cook for an additional 5 minutes.
6. Serve hot.

TIPS:

- Adjust the amount of cayenne pepper to your preferred spice level.
- Serve with a dollop of Greek yogurt to balance the heat.

NUTRITIONAL VALUES: Calories: 220, Fat: 4g, Carbs: 36g, Protein: 12g, Sugar: 6g

Creamy Broccoli and Cauliflower Soup

PREPARATION TIME: 10 min
COOKING TIME: 25 min
MODE OF COOKING: Simmering and Blending

INGREDIENTS:

- 2 Tbsp olive oil
- 1 onion, diced
- 2 cloves garlic, minced
- 4 cups broccoli florets
- 4 cups cauliflower florets
- 4 cups vegetable broth
- 1 cup unsweetened almond milk
- Salt and pepper to taste

DIRECTIONS:

1. In a large pot, heat olive oil over medium heat. Add onion and garlic, sauté until softened.
2. Add broccoli and cauliflower, cook for 5 minutes.
3. Stir in vegetable broth, bring to a boil.
4. Reduce heat and simmer for 20 minutes, until vegetables are tender.
5. Using an immersion blender, blend the soup until smooth. Stir in almond milk.
6. Season with salt and pepper to taste and serve hot.

TIPS:

- Garnish with chopped chives or a sprinkle of cheddar cheese.
- Serve with a side salad for a light meal.

NUTRITIONAL VALUES: Calories: 180, Fat: 9g, Carbs: 20g, Protein: 5g, Sugar: 4g

Moroccan Chickpea Stew

PREPARATION TIME: 15 min
COOKING TIME: 35 min
MODE OF COOKING: Simmering
INGREDIENTS:

- 2 Tbsp olive oil
- 1 onion, diced
- 3 cloves garlic, minced
- 1 tsp ginger, minced
- 1 tsp cumin
- 1 tsp cinnamon
- 1 tsp paprika
- 1/2 tsp cayenne pepper
- 1 can diced tomatoes
- 4 cups vegetable broth
- 2 cans chickpeas, rinsed and drained
- 2 cups butternut squash, diced
- 1/4 cup dried apricots, chopped
- Salt and pepper to taste

DIRECTIONS:

1. In a large pot, heat olive oil over medium heat. Add onion, garlic, and ginger, sauté until softened.
2. Stir in cumin, cinnamon, paprika, and cayenne pepper, cook for 1 minute.
3. Add diced tomatoes, vegetable broth, chickpeas, butternut squash, and dried apricots. Bring to a boil.
4. Reduce heat and simmer for 30 minutes, until squash is tender.
5. Season with salt and pepper to taste and serve hot.

TIPS:

- Serve over couscous or quinoa for a heartier meal.
- Garnish with fresh cilantro and a squeeze of lemon juice.

NUTRITIONAL VALUES: Calories: 280, Fat: 8g, Carbs: 44g, Protein: 10g, Sugar: 10g

Tomato Basil Soup

PREPARATION TIME: 10 min
COOKING TIME: 25 min
MODE OF COOKING: Simmering
INGREDIENTS:

- 2 Tbsp olive oil
- 1 onion, diced
- 3 cloves garlic, minced
- 2 cans diced tomatoes
- 4 cups vegetable broth
- 1/4 cup fresh basil, chopped
- 1 tsp dried oregano
- 1 cup unsweetened almond milk
- Salt and pepper to taste

DIRECTIONS:

1. In a large pot, heat olive oil over medium heat. Add onion and garlic, sauté until softened.
2. Stir in diced tomatoes, vegetable broth, basil, and oregano. Bring to a boil.
3. Reduce heat and simmer for 20 minutes.

4. Using an immersion blender, blend the soup until smooth. Stir in almond milk.
5. Season with salt and pepper to taste and serve hot.

TIPS:
- Garnish with fresh basil leaves and a drizzle of olive oil.
- Serve with a grilled cheese sandwich for a classic pairing.

NUTRITIONAL VALUES: Calories: 160, Fat: 7g, Carbs: 22g, Protein: 3g, Sugar: 10g

BUTTERNUT SQUASH SOUP

PREPARATION TIME: 15 min
COOKING TIME: 30 min
MODE OF COOKING: Simmering and Blending
INGREDIENTS:
- 2 Tbsp olive oil
- 1 onion, diced
- 3 cloves garlic, minced
- 4 cups butternut squash, peeled and diced
- 4 cups vegetable broth
- 1 cup coconut milk
- 1 tsp ground nutmeg
- Salt and pepper to taste

DIRECTIONS:
1. In a large pot, heat olive oil over medium heat. Add onion and garlic, sauté until softened.
2. Add butternut squash and vegetable broth, bring to a boil.
3. Reduce heat and simmer for 25 minutes, until squash is tender.
4. Using an immersion blender, blend the soup until smooth. Stir in coconut milk and nutmeg.
5. Season with salt and pepper to taste and serve hot.

TIPS:
- Garnish with roasted pumpkin seeds or a sprinkle of cinnamon.
- Serve with a side of crusty bread.

NUTRITIONAL VALUES: Calories: 200, Fat: 10g, Carbs: 28g, Protein: 3g, Sugar: 6g

MUSHROOM BARLEY SOUP

PREPARATION TIME: 15 min
COOKING TIME: 40 min
MODE OF COOKING: Simmering
INGREDIENTS:
- 2 Tbsp olive oil
- 1 onion, diced
- 2 cloves garlic, minced
- 2 cups mushrooms, sliced
- 1 cup barley
- 4 cups vegetable broth

- 1 cup carrots, diced
- 1 cup celery, diced
- 1 tsp dried thyme
- Salt and pepper to taste

DIRECTIONS:
1. In a large pot, heat olive oil over medium heat. Add onion and garlic, sauté until softened.
2. Add mushrooms and cook for 5 minutes, until tender.
3. Stir in barley, vegetable broth, carrots, celery, and thyme. Bring to a boil.
4. Reduce heat and simmer for 30 minutes, until barley is tender.
5. Season with salt and pepper to taste and serve hot.

TIPS:
- Garnish with fresh parsley.
- Serve with a side salad for a complete meal.

NUTRITIONAL VALUES: Calories: 240, Fat: 8g, Carbs: 38g, Protein: 6g, Sugar: 6g

SWEET POTATO AND BLACK BEAN CHILI

PREPARATION TIME: 15 min
COOKING TIME: 40 min
MODE OF COOKING: Simmering
INGREDIENTS:
- 2 Tbsp olive oil
- 1 onion, diced
- 3 cloves garlic, minced
- 1 red bell pepper, diced
- 2 medium sweet potatoes, diced
- 1 can diced tomatoes
- 4 cups vegetable broth
- 2 cans black beans, rinsed and drained
- 1 Tbsp chili powder
- 1 tsp cumin
- 1 tsp smoked paprika
- Salt and pepper to taste

DIRECTIONS:
1. In a large pot, heat olive oil over medium heat. Add onion and garlic, sauté until softened.
2. Add red bell pepper and sweet potatoes, cook for 5 minutes.
3. Stir in diced tomatoes, vegetable broth, black beans, chili powder, cumin, smoked paprika, salt, and pepper. Bring to a boil.
4. Reduce heat and simmer for 30 minutes, until sweet potatoes are tender.
5. Serve hot.

TIPS:
- Garnish with avocado slices and fresh cilantro.
- Serve with cornbread for a hearty meal.

NUTRITIONAL VALUES: Calories: 280, Fat: 6g, Carbs: 48g, Protein: 10g, Sugar: 10g

Minestrone Soup

PREPARATION TIME: 15 min
COOKING TIME: 30 min
MODE OF COOKING: Simmering
INGREDIENTS:

- 2 Tbsp olive oil
- 1 onion, diced
- 3 cloves garlic, minced
- 2 carrots, diced
- 2 celery stalks, diced
- 1 zucchini, diced
- 1 can diced tomatoes
- 4 cups vegetable broth
- 1 can kidney beans, rinsed and drained
- 1 cup small pasta (like ditalini)
- 1 tsp dried basil
- 1 tsp dried oregano
- Salt and pepper to taste

DIRECTIONS:

1. In a large pot, heat olive oil over medium heat. Add onion and garlic, sauté until softened.
2. Add carrots, celery, and zucchini, cook for 5 minutes.
3. Stir in diced tomatoes, vegetable broth, kidney beans, pasta, basil, oregano, salt, and pepper. Bring to a boil.
4. Reduce heat and simmer for 20 minutes, until pasta is tender.
5. Serve hot.

TIPS:

- Garnish with grated Parmesan cheese.
- Serve with a side of garlic bread.

NUTRITIONAL VALUES: Calories: 240, Fat: 7g, Carbs: 38g, Protein: 8g, Sugar: 8g

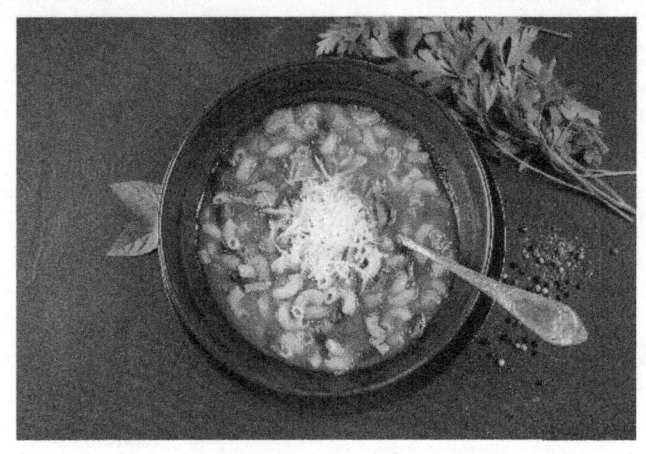

Coconut Curry Soup

PREPARATION TIME: 10 min
COOKING TIME: 20 min
MODE OF COOKING: Simmering
INGREDIENTS:

- 1 Tbsp olive oil
- 1 onion, diced
- 2 cloves garlic, minced
- 1 Tbsp ginger, minced
- 1 Tbsp red curry paste
- 4 cups vegetable broth
- 1 can coconut milk
- 1 cup carrots, sliced
- 1 red bell pepper, sliced
- 1 cup mushrooms, sliced
- 2 cups spinach, chopped
- 1 Tbsp lime juice
- Salt and pepper to taste

DIRECTIONS:
1. In a large pot, heat olive oil over medium heat. Add onion, garlic, and ginger, sauté until softened.
2. Stir in red curry paste and cook for 1 minute.
3. Add vegetable broth, coconut milk, carrots, red bell pepper, and mushrooms. Bring to a boil.
4. Reduce heat and simmer for 15 minutes, until vegetables are tender.
5. Stir in spinach and lime juice, cook for an additional 2 minutes.
6. Season with salt and pepper to taste and serve hot.

TIPS:
- Garnish with fresh cilantro and a lime wedge.
- Serve with jasmine rice or naan bread.

NUTRITIONAL VALUES: Calories: 230, Fat: 15g, Carbs: 20g, Protein: 4g, Sugar: 6g

MEASUREMENT CONVERSION TABLE

Volume Conversions

Volume (Liquid)	US Customary Units	Metric Units
1 teaspoon	1 tsp	5 milliliters (ml)
1 tablespoon	1 tbsp	15 milliliters
1 fluid ounce	1 fl oz	30 milliliters
1 cup	1 cup	240 milliliters
1 pint	1 pt	473 milliliters
1 quart	1 qt	946 milliliters
1 gallon	1 gal	3.785 liters

Weight Conversions

Weight	US Customary Units	Metric Units
1 ounce	1 oz	28 grams (g)
1 pound	1 lb	454 grams
1 kilogram	2.2 lbs	1000 grams (1 kg)

Length Conversions

Length	US Customary Units	Metric Units
1 inch	1 in	2.54 centimeters (cm)
1 foot	1 ft	30.48 centimeters

Metric Volume Conversions

Volume	Metric Units	US Customary Units
1 milliliter (ml)	1 ml	0.034 fluid ounce (fl oz)
100 milliliters	100 ml	3.4 fluid ounces
1 liter (L)	1 L	34 fluid ounces
		4.2 cups
		2.1 pints
		1.06 quarts
		0.26 gallon

Metric Weight Conversions

Weight	Metric Units	US Customary Units
1 gram (g)	1 g	0.035 ounces (oz)
100 grams	100 g	3.5 ounces
500 grams	500 g	1.1 pounds (lb)
1 kilogram (kg)	1 kg	2.2 pounds

Temperature Conversions

Temperature	Celsius (°C)	Fahrenheit (°F)
Freezing Point	0°C	32°F
Refrigerator	4°C	39°F
Room Temperature	20°C - 22°C	68°F - 72°F
Boiling Water	100°C	212°F

CHAPTER 14: WHAT TO EAT WHEN YOU'RE OUT

Navigating the landscape of dining out while adhering to the Galveston Diet can seem daunting at first, but with a little foresight and some strategic choices, you can enjoy delicious meals without compromising your health goals. Eating out is a delightful social experience, and you should feel empowered to partake without worry. Here's how to do it with confidence and ease.

First and foremost, preparation is key. Before heading out to a restaurant, take a moment to check the menu online. Many restaurants provide their menus on their websites, complete with nutritional information. This allows you to make informed choices and plan your meal ahead of time. If the nutritional information isn't available, look for dishes that emphasize whole, minimally processed foods.

When scanning the menu, focus on dishes that highlight lean proteins, vegetables, and healthy fats. Opt for grilled, baked, or steamed proteins like chicken, fish, or tofu rather than fried or breaded options. For example, a grilled salmon dish with a side of steamed vegetables or a salad is a fantastic choice that aligns well with the principles of the Galveston Diet. Avoid creamy sauces and opt for lighter options like vinaigrettes or olive oil and lemon juice.

Salads are often a safe bet, but be cautious of hidden calories in dressings and toppings. Ask for dressing on the side, and choose olive oil and vinegar over creamy dressings. Load up on vegetables and lean proteins, and skip high-calorie extras like croutons and cheese. A salad with mixed greens, grilled chicken, avocado, and a variety of fresh vegetables can be both satisfying and nourishing.

If you're in the mood for something heartier, look for entrée options that feature a balance of protein, vegetables, and whole grains. Many restaurants now offer bowls that combine these elements beautifully. A quinoa bowl with grilled shrimp, roasted vegetables, and a light tahini dressing can be a delicious and nutritious option. Remember to request modifications if needed—most restaurants are happy to accommodate dietary preferences.

Portion control is another important aspect to consider. Restaurant portions are often larger than necessary, so don't hesitate to ask for a half-portion or to box up half of your meal right away. This way, you can enjoy your meal without overeating and have leftovers for the next day.

When it comes to beverages, water is always a safe and healthy choice. If you prefer something with a bit more flavor, unsweetened iced tea or sparkling water with a slice of lemon or lime are excellent alternatives. Avoid sugary drinks and alcohol, as they can add unnecessary calories and disrupt your dietary goals. If you do choose to drink alcohol, opt for a glass of dry wine and enjoy it slowly. Dessert can be tempting, but it's often loaded with sugar and unhealthy fats. If you're craving something sweet, look for fruit-based options or share a dessert with someone.

Fresh berries with a dollop of whipped cream or a fruit sorbet can satisfy your sweet tooth without derailing your diet. Alternatively, consider bringing a small piece of dark chocolate with you to enjoy after your meal.

Buffets and social gatherings can present additional challenges, but they are manageable with a strategic approach. Start by surveying all the options available and make a mental plan. Fill your plate with a variety of vegetables and lean proteins first. Avoid fried foods, heavy sauces, and sugary desserts. A plate filled with a colorful array of vegetables, grilled meats, and perhaps a small portion of whole grains is both satisfying and aligned with your dietary goals.

Eating out should be an enjoyable experience, not a source of stress. Remember that you have the power to make choices that support your health and well-being. By focusing on whole, minimally processed foods, controlling portions, and making mindful choices, you can dine out confidently and maintain your commitment to the Galveston Diet.

Moreover, don't be afraid to communicate your needs to the restaurant staff. Politely asking for modifications to your meal is completely acceptable and ensures that you get exactly what you need. Whether it's substituting a side of fries with a side salad or requesting no butter on your steamed vegetables, most restaurants are more than willing to accommodate.

It's also helpful to have a few go-to restaurants that you know offer healthy options. Over time, you'll become familiar with the menus and the best choices available, making dining out even easier. Additionally, exploring new cuisines can be a fun and healthful adventure. Mediterranean, Japanese, and Thai cuisines, for instance, often feature dishes that are naturally aligned with the principles of the Galveston Diet.

When dining at a friend's or family member's home, offer to bring a dish that fits within your dietary guidelines. This not only ensures there's something you can enjoy but also introduces others to delicious, healthy options. Sharing recipes and tips can also be a great way to inspire others to join you in your healthy eating journey.

Ultimately, the goal is to enjoy your meals and the company you're with while staying true to your health goals. The Galveston Diet is about fostering a lifestyle that supports hormonal balance, reduces inflammation, and enhances overall well-being. With these strategies in place, you can savor the experience of eating out, knowing that you're making choices that nourish your body and support your long-term health.

Dining out should be a pleasure, a time to relax and enjoy good food and good company. By planning ahead, making mindful choices, and not being afraid to ask for what you need, you can enjoy all the social and culinary benefits of dining out while staying true to your dietary goals. Embrace the journey and enjoy the delicious possibilities that await you.

28 DAYS EASY MEAL PLAN

WEEK 1-2	breakfast	snack	lunch	snack	dinner
Monday	Avocado and Smoked Salmon Breakfast Bowl	Spicy Roasted Chickpeas	Grilled Chicken and Quinoa Salad	Roasted Brussels Sprouts with Balsamic Glaze	Lemon Herb Grilled Salmon
Tuesday	Spinach and Mushroom Frittata	Greek Yogurt and Cucumber Dip	Turkey and Avocado Lettuce Wraps	Garlic Parmesan Kale Chips	Baked Chicken with Asparagus and Tomatoes
Wednesday	Greek Yogurt Parfait with Berries and Nuts	Baked Zucchini Fries	Spinach and Feta Stuffed Peppers	Guacamole and Veggie Sticks	Beef and Broccoli Stir-Fry
Thursday	Chia Seed Pudding with Almond Milk	Avocado Deviled Eggs	Mediterranean Chickpea Salad	Greek Yogurt with Fresh Berries	Shrimp and Avocado Salad
Friday	Vegetable and Egg Breakfast Muffins	Garlic and Herb Cauliflower Mash	Grilled Shrimp Tacos with Avocado Salsa	Mixed Nuts and Seeds	Lemon Garlic Chicken Thighs
Saturday	Quinoa Breakfast Bowl	Spicy Edamame	Chicken and Vegetable Stir-Fry	Cucumber Slices with Hummus	Stuffed Bell Peppers with Turkey and Quinoa
Sunday	Sweet Potato and Avocado Toast	Sweet Potato Chips	Tuna and White Bean Salad	Apple Slices with Almond Butter	Balsamic Glazed Pork Chops

WEEK 3-4	breakfast	snack	lunch	snack	dinner
Monday	Almond Butter and Banana Smoothie	Berry Chia Pudding	Lentil and Kale Soup	Tomato Basil Soup	Blackened Salmon
Tuesday	Savory Oatmeal with Spinach and Egg	Almond Butter Banana Bites	Balsamic Chicken and Veggie Skewers	Butternut Squash Soup	Baked Tilapia with Cherry Tomatoes
Wednesday	Coconut Yogurt with Pineapple and Almonds	Coconut Macaroons	Quinoa and Black Bean Stuffed Sweet Potatoes	Mushroom Barley Soup	Grilled Mahi with Pineapple Salsa
Thursday	Avocado and Tomato on Toast	Greek Yogurt and Berry Popsicles	Tuscan White Bean Soup	Sweet Potato and Black Bean Chili	Seared Scallops with Lemon Garlic Butter
Friday	Scrambled Tofu with Vegetables	Dark Chocolate and Almond Clusters	Spicy Lentil Stew	Minestrone Soup	Honey Lime Glazed Shrimp
Saturday	Berry Smoothie Bowl	Baked Apple Chips	Creamy Broccoli and Cauliflower Soup	Coconut Curry Soup	Baked Lemon Dill Halibut
Sunday	Mushroom and Spinach Omelet	Lemon Blueberry Muffins	Moroccan Chickpea Stew	Fresh Veggies with Hummus	Cajun Catfish with Red Pepper Aioli

THANK YOU FOR READING

Dear Reader,

Thank you so much for purchasing my book! I sincerely hope it provides you with both enjoyment and inspiration. Your support plays a pivotal role in my journey as an author.

If you could spare a few moments to leave a review, I would greatly appreciate it. Your insights help me to grow and improve, and they aid other readers in choosing their next book.

As a small expression of my gratitude, I invite you to scan the QR code below to access exclusive bonus content available just for you.

Warmest thanks once again for your support.

Best regards,

Marie Dowson

Made in the USA
Coppell, TX
15 May 2025